Who's **Who** in *Dogs*

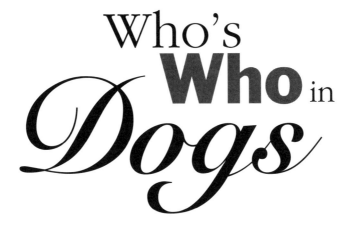

Who's Who in Dogs

Connie Vanacore

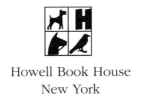

Howell Book House
New York

Howell Book House
A Simon & Schuster Macmillan Company
1633 Broadway
New York, NY 10019

Macmillan Publishing books may be purchased for business or sales promotional use. For informantion please write: Special Markets Department, Macmillan Publishing USA, 1633 Broadway, New York, NY 10019.

Library of Congress Cataloging-in-Publication Data

Vanacore, Connie.
    Who's who in dogs / Connie Vanacore.
        p.   cm.
    ISBN 0-87605-591-9
    1. Dog specialists—United States—Biography—Dictionaries.
  I. Title.
  SF422.8.U6V35   1997   97-30075
  636.7'0092'273—dc21   CIP

Manufactured in the United States of America

10 9 8 7 6 5 4 3 2 1

To all those who encouraged me to write this book and to my husband, Fred, who took up the burdens on the home front to give me the time to devote to it.

Contents

There are no entries in this book for Q, U, and X.

Acknowledgments

We are grateful for the help we have received in compiling this book. We appreciate the time given by all those who responded to our request for information about themselves.

We are especially indebted to the staff of the American Kennel Club Library and those within AKC who have contributed names and information to us. To Barbara Kolk and Ann Sergi at the Library we owe a special thank-you.

Our research into individual breed books provided us additional material, as did the wonderful book of reminiscences, *My Times With Dogs,* by the dean of dog writers, Walter Fletcher.

There is a wealth of information out there about dogs and the people who love them. Thanks to everyone who made this book possible.

Introduction

A book about people involved in dogs is a work in progress. It is never complete because of the ebb and flow of interest in the sport of dogs. To include everyone who has made a contribution to our sport one would have to start at the beginning when breeders first took one dog to another in order to enhance some particular trait. We would have to go back to ancient Egypt to those keepers of the pharoahs' dogs, or to China's emperors. More recently we could look to Parson Jack Russell and his dauntless terriers, to Mr. Llewellyn or Mr. Laverack whose breeding programs designed the English Setter as we know it today.

Every breeder who ever designed a litter with the ambition of improving the breed belongs in this book. Every person who ever contributed time, energy, money, resources and goodwill in the process of forming a dog club, putting on a show, field trial, obedience trial, lure coursing, agility or earth dog event belongs in this book. Every veterinarian who treated a pet, designed a vaccine, saved a dog's life, ran a spay clinic or sat in the rain under the tent at a dog show belongs in this book.

The 4-H families who foster guide dogs, volunteers who bring their dogs to fairs, parades, nursing homes, schools to teach others about purebred dogs and responsible dog ownership deserve a line in this book. Every person, from field rep to the Chairman of the Board of AKC belongs in a *Who's Who In Dogs*.

Where does that leave the poor compiler of names? We obviously cannot list them all and there will be, without any doubt, those worthy individuals who should have been included, but whose names are missing. As mightily as we tried to include representatives of every breed, we have come up short. This should come as no surprise, given the nature of clubs and their personnel, but now that the book is a published reality, there are bound to be some disappointed souls. We apologize to those whose names have been omitted. We admit that this book could easily have remained unfinished until the end of time, as we gathered additional people into the fold.

The nature of the sport of purebred dogs is that those who participate over a long period of time are far outnumbered by those who are in it for two or three years, sometimes as long as a decade. There are really a small number who have made lasting and significant contributions. We have attempted, to the best of our ability, to include all or most of them. Some of those listed in this compendium are no longer with us, but they live on in our collective memories. They are here because we consider them to have been significant participants in some aspect of the sport. Their experience and wisdom has survived through those who have followed in their paths.

This is an idiosyncratic book. People appear because of the perception of the author that they belong. Others do not appear because requested information about them is lacking. For those omissions, we are truly sorry. Where possible the biographies are written in the language submitted by those who sent their own information. That is the reason for the variable format, but we thought it would make for more interesting reading.

We were particularly struck by the diversity of interests and backgrounds of many of our biographies and we were moved by the number of people who served in the armed forces at some point in their lives.

It is our hope that by learning a little of the background and experience of those people included in this unfinished work, you who read about them will gain inspiration to achieve your own goals.

Connie Vanacore

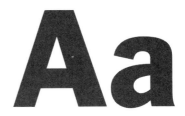

AGUIRRE, GUSTAVO, VMD, PhD, PhD hc. Gustavo Aguirre earned his undergraduate, professional and graduate degrees at the University of Pennsylvania. He joined the University of Pennsylvania as an assistant professor of ophthalmology in 1973, rose to hold joint professorships in ophthalmology at the Veterinary and Medical Schools and served as director of the Inherited Eye Disease Studies Unit. In 1992 he joined Cornell University's Baker Institute for Animal Health, where he heads the Center for Canine Genetics and Reproduction, a division of the institute.

Dr. Aguirre served as president of the International Society of Veterinary Ophthalmology from 1986 to 1989. In 1993 he received an honorary doctorate from the University of Goteborg, Sweden, and in 1996, the American Veterinary Medical Association awarded him the AKC Excellence in Canine Research award.

Dr. Aguirre's research is focused on inherited eye diseases, particularly those that affect the retina. He has identified the major diseases grouped under the term Progressive Retinal Atrophy (PRA) and has pioneered their early diagnosis, using electroretinography. More recently, his interests have focused on the molecular biology and genetics of these disorders. His research group has identified the mutation that causes the rod cone dysplasia form of PRA in Irish Setters and developed a blood-based DNA test to identify genetically normal carriers and affected dogs.

ALSTON, GEORGE. George Alston grew up with Boxers, which his mother bred and raised. He was in the show ring before he became a teen and was best Junior handler at Westminster in 1954, one of the youngest to ever achieve that success. He apprenticed to a series of the greatest professional handlers in the conformation sport before embarking on his own successful career. He was a Quaker Oats award winner several times with dogs he piloted for his clients. Alston began teaching handling classes in the 1970s, and since his retirement from professional handling he has traveled the country, giving seminars and classes. He is a master teacher and particularly enjoys guiding the youngsters who take his courses.

In addition to his classes, Alston is president of K-9 Bytes, a computer software company that he founded to serve the dog Fancy. He is also the author of a book, written with Connie Vanacore, *The Winning Edge, Show Ring Secrets* (New York: Howell Book House, 1992).

He has four children, one of whom, Lisa Jane Alston-Myers, handled the Clumber Spaniel Ch. Clussex Country Sunrise to Best in Show at the 1996 Westminster KC show, following in her father's footsteps as a professional handler.

ALSTON, MARY ANN. As with her husband, George, Mary Ann Alston showed dogs as a teen. She was raised on a game farm where her father was the gamekeeper, and her first dog was an English Setter that she showed to its championship. She did not enter the ranks of the professional handlers until much later, after she completed college and began a career as a teacher.

She met George on the show circuit, and eventually they both apprenticed to Bill Trainor. After they married and moved to Maryland they embarked on careers as one of the most successful handling couples in the business for more than twenty-five years.

Mary Ann Alston was a successful breeder of English Cocker and English Springer Spaniels, Irish, English and Gordon Setters. She now has turned her expertise to rare cat breeds. She is an AKC-approved judge of all Sporting breeds and most of the Hound Group.

ANDERSON, SHARON. Sharon Anderson is AKC Agility field director. She started in Obedience in 1969, when she put a CD on her German Shepherd Dog. Since that modest beginning she has earned many Obedience titles, including several OTCHs. She has belonged to a number of kennel clubs and served as Obedience Trial chairwoman on several occasions. In the 1980s Anderson became interested in Agility and started a club in her home state of Minnesota, which became the largest Agility club in the United States. In 1993 she was invited to be on the Agility Advisory Committee by the AKC. In 1994 she became Agility consultant to the Events Department and subsequently became Agility director.

ANSELM, DR. KLAUS. Dr. Anselm, a gastroenterologist from Beulah, Colorado, breeds Giant Schnauzers, which he shows in conformation and Obedience competition. He and his wife, Joan, have been active in local all-breed clubs and in the Giant Schnauzer Club of America. Dr. Anselm is a delegate to the American Kennel Club from the Southern Colorado Kennel Club. He judges all Working breeds and half the breeds in the Sporting Group.

ANTYPAS, CARMEN VISSER. Her first love being music, Carmen Antypas was sidetracked into dog shows through the enthusiasm of Jack Bradshaw Jr. while she worked for his superintending organization in the late 1960s and 1970s. At this time she began a friendship with Mr. and Mrs. Tom Stevenson of the Santa Barbara Kennel Club that has resulted in her playing a key role as secretary-treasurer of this club. In turn, the Santa Barbara Kennel Club was influential in her career. The first show Ms. Antypas superintended was the 4,445 dog–Santa Barbara Kennel Club show in July 1975 with her former husband, Neal Visser.

In 1981 she and Bill Antypas founded Newport Dog Shows, a non-profit California corporation. She has also been the guiding inspiration for the World competition in Junior Showmanship, which is sponsored by Pedigree foods.

ANTYPAS, DR. WILLIAM G. Dr. Antypas received his undergraduate degree from Williams College in Massachusetts. He spent a year on a special project with Monsanto Chemical Company. On completion of this project Dr. Antypas entered the California Institute of Technology, where he received his PhD in biochemistry. Concurrently he established the Mosbour Corporation and Newport Dog Shows. He is the American Kennel Club principal licensed superintendent for Newport Dog Shows, a position he has held since 1981.

Dr. Antypas serves as the resident computer specialist for both Mosbour Corporation and Newport Dog Shows and does consulting in software management and chemistry. His hobbies include restoring vintage British motorcars.

APPEL, MAX J., DVM, PhD. Dr. Appel is professor of Virology at the James A. Baker Institute for Animal Health at the College of Veterinary Medicine, Cornell University in Ithaca, New York. He received his degree in veterinary medicine in 1956 from the College of Veterinary Medicine, Hannover, Germany, and his PhD from Cornell University in 1967.

During his thirty-year tenure at the Baker Institute he has devoted the majority of his research toward the study and prevention of canine infectious diseases. He was first to isolate canine parvovirus in 1978 and, together with Dr. Leland Carmichael, developed vaccines to protect dogs against infection. Both investigators were also responsible for the shift from CAV-1 (ICH) to CAV-2 vaccines for dogs, which prevented "blue eyes" and other side reactions in dogs. Dr. Appel is a specialist for canine distemper. He is now involved in research in Lyme disease in

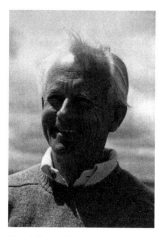

Max J. Appel, DVM, PhD, professor of Virology, James A. Baker Institute for Animal Health.

dogs, including prevention by vaccination and treatment.

Dr. Appel is married to Barbara Hocke. They have four children and live in Ithaca, New York.

ARCHIBALD, JOHN. John Archibald, with his wife, Margie, was a guiding force in the American Boxer Club from 1948 until his death in 1981. He was chairman of the National Specialty show for twelve years and brought it from a small regional show to an enormously successful weeklong event. He served in many other capacities, including president of the national club. He was the club's delegate to the AKC until his death.

ARCHIBALD, MARGARET. Together with her husband, John, Margie Archibald was a tireless worker and guiding influence in the American Boxer Club. Upon her husband's death she assumed his duties as show chairwoman, the first woman to hold that post, and she was also the first woman president of the club. She is currently the club's AKC delegate.

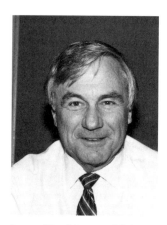

Lorenz "Don" Arner, publisher.

ARNER, LORENZ "DON". Don Arner is as versatile a person in training, Obedience work and communications as one could find. He was the cofounder and an officer in the Adirondack Search and Rescue Dog Association, American Rescue Dog Association and the International Federation of Rescue Dog Associations. He developed prototype programs for research and government agencies to use dogs for pollutant, insect and agricultural detection. He trained bears for game farms and developed the Beagle Brigade concept for the United States Department of Agriculture (USDA). He has instructed fourteen dog handlers to AKC Tracking titles without a failure. He is past director of the German Shepherd Dog Club and its Working Dog Association. He has trained several German Shepherd Dogs to Schutzhund degrees and AKC titles.

Arner is the founder of the largest boarding, grooming and training facility in New York State and is a charter member of the American Boarding Kennel Association. He is the founder and editor of *Off-Lead,* a monthly publication for dog training instructors.

He served as manager of Professional Markets for Hills Pet Nutrition and is an international lecturer on pet care and training. He is also the winner of several awards for his writing.

In his spare time, Don Arner enjoys photography, sailing and gardening.

AUBREY-JONES, NIGEL. Nigel is the consummate "dog person." For the past forty years he has judged, bred, sold or owned dogs of various breeds that have won more than 800 Best in Show awards, including two Westminster Best in Show winners (1960, 1982). The Pekingese, Int. Ch. Chik T'Sun of Caversham, imported from England by Jones was, for a number of years, the world record holder of BIS wins in the United States with 139 top awards.

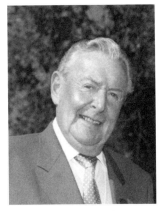

His judging career spans the globe from Europe to Asia. He has officiated at Crufts in England and at shows in Hong Kong and Thailand.

Nigel Aubrey-Jones, writer, international judge, importer, breeder and owner of Bibliography of the Dog.

He is a prolific writer for dog magazines and newspapers and is the author of *The New Pekingese* (New York: Howell Book House, 1990). Although semiretired, he devotes time to his unique business, the Bibliography of the Dog. He handles only dog-related oil paintings, bronzes, porcelains, prints and books originating before 1940.

Although primarily associated with Pekingese, Nigel Aubrey-Jones also was successful with an imported Greyhound and a Whippet, Ch. Charmol Clansman, which he bought for the late James Butt.

Bb

BALDWIN, DYANE. Dyane Baldwin's kennel, Pond Hollow, has produced Chesapeake Bay Retrievers that have been recognized as significant winners and producers influential in the breed. She has served as chairwoman of the AKC-American Chesapeake Club video project and was the club's Judge's Education coordinator for ten years. She was chairwoman of the illustrated judging guide project and is currently the club historian and editor of the upcoming American Chesapeake Club breed book. She has spearheaded efforts to educate breeders and the public about progressive retinal atrophy in the Chesapeake Bay Retriever.

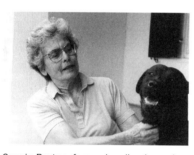

Connie Barton, former handler, kennel manager and AKC field representative with a favorite Labrador Retriever.

BARTON, CONSTANCE. Connie Barton showed a Doberman Pinscher in the late 1940s and had a few litters. This hobby turned into a long road of activities involving dogs.

About ten years later she became a professional handler, with the added responsibility of importing dogs and planning breeding programs for clients.

In the 1960s she ran a successful show and breeding kennel, Springfield, owned by Elizabeth Clark, concentrating on Labrador Retrievers and some terrier breeds.

In the mid-1970s she was pleased to join the AKC as a field representative and for the next sixteen years enjoyed another part of the dog world.

Connie gave up her position in order to become a judge and is now approved for all Sporting, Hound and Working breeds.

Needlepoint has been a relaxing hobby, and gardening also rates high on her list of things she loves to do.

Her eldest daughter, Deborah Ayer, has her involved in the showing and breeding of Cavalier King Charles Spaniels. She will be another generation of "dog" people.

BASQUETTE, LINA. Surely one of the most colorful characters in all of dogdom was the legendary actress and Great Dane breeder, handler and judge, Lina Basquette. Famous for her roles in silent movies in the late 1920s and 1930s, as well as a stint on Broadway as one of the Ziegfield girls, Basquette was equally renown for her off-screen antics. She was married nine times to seven different husbands, the first of whom was Sam Warner, founder of Warner Brothers film studio.

Her show-business career was marked by tempestuous highs and lows, punctuated by several suicide attempts and lurid affairs. When talking films took over, Lina Basquette's movie career was effectively over, although from time to time she garnered roles, the last of which was in the 1991 film *Paradise Park*.

In 1947 Basquette began a second career as a breeder and handler of Great Danes. Her Honey Hollow Kennels in Bucks County, Pennsylvania, produced nearly 100 titleholders, the most famous of which was Special-K, a bitch who broke all records for the breed. Basquette was licensed to judge all Working breeds, Junior showmanship and Best in Show, and she made as much of a statement in the center of the ring as she did as a handler or a showgirl. She died in 1994 at the age of eighty-seven.

BATTAGLIA, DR. CARMEN. German Shepherd Dogs have been Carmen's abiding interest for many years. He has worked within the German Shepherd Dog Club of America to improve the health of the breed by recognition of sound hips and elbows and by advocating the total dog. Under his guidance as president of the national club each National Specialty must offer conformation, Obedience, Herding, Tracking and Agility events.

Carmen is the GSDCA's delegate to the American Kennel Club and serves on AKC's board of directors. He is a nationally recognized author and lecturer on dog genetics and methods of breeding better dogs. He regularly contributes articles to several dog-related publications.

Professionally, he is a consultant in the educational field and has written a book about disadvantaged students. He is a lecturer and commencement speaker at schools throughout the country.

BAUER, RICHARD. Richard Bauer was born in New York City in 1938 and attended school in Manhattan. He started his long, illustrious career in dogs at the age of thirteen with a white Boxer named "Duke." Bauer spent a lot of time with Duke in Central Park, basking in the sun in the hopes that Duke would eventually turn tan! Richard did get a leg toward a Utility title between sun rays.

The next breed with which he was associated was the Papillion. His Admiral of Mariposa, UDT was the Obedience Dog of the Year in 1955.

After returning from military service at age eighteen, Richard Bauer attended the Morris and Essex show, hovering around Anne Hone Rogers and Jane Kamp (later Clark and Forsyth, respectively). At one point, Bauer recalls, Janie said, "Hey, kid. If you run real quick and tell Annie she has to show a dog for me in the Sporting Group, I'll let you hold 'Barrage' for me." That was the great-winning Boxer of the day, Ch. Barrage of Quality Hill. That errand was the beginning of a long association with Mrs. Clark that lasted more than ten years.

Acting as Mrs. Clark's assistant, Bauer was exposed to many of the top dogs of the day. Because of his solid grounding and experience, he reaped great success in the show ring and was able to pilot many of Mrs. Clark's charges to Best in Show awards. When his employer married James Clark in 1965 and retired as a handler, Bauer successfully took over her kennel in Mahopac, New York. He continued to handle for more than twenty-five years, becoming one of the country's top professionals.

He retired from handling in September 1991 and has since been a sought-after judge of the Terrier and Toy Non-Sporting Groups, as well as fifteen additional breeds in other Groups.

BEAUCHAMP, RICHARD G. Rick Beauchamp was raised with field dogs in the Midwest—Irish and English Setters and Beagles. As a teenager he chose American Cocker Spaniels to breed and exhibit.

Since then he has been successfully involved in practically every facet of purebred dogs; breeding, exhibiting, professional handling, publishing, writing and judging. He has assisted in writing the official breed Standards for several breeds and has lectured extensively throughout the world.

After moving to California in 1962 Rick purchased the local southern California magazine, *Kennel Review*, and developed it into one of the leading breeder-exhibitor magazines in the world. As the publisher, Rick involved serious exhibitors, breeders and handlers with his concept of recognizing the top people in the Fancy. He instituted the *Kennel Review* annual awards that were presented at gala events annually for several years. Recipients often list these credentials with great pride.

He is a prolific writer, is published in dog periodicals throughout the world and is the author of several breed books.

As a breeder-exhibitor himself Rick has been actively involved in many different breeds. Among these are Chow Chows, Dachshunds, Salukis and Irish Setters. His Beau Monde Kennel has produced outstanding Boxers,

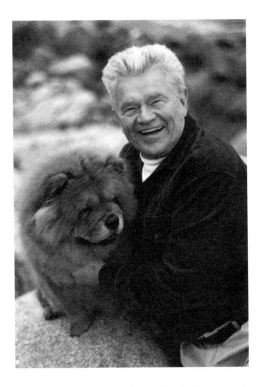

Richard Beauchamp, publisher, writer, judge, breeder.

American Cocker Spaniels, Poodles, Wire Fox Terriers, Bull Terriers, Pembroke Welsh Corgis, Cavalier King Charles Spaniels and Chinese Shar-Pei.

He was instrumental in achieving American Kennel Club recognition for the Bichon Frise in the early 1970s and has bred more than sixty champion Bichons himself. Many of the current winners in the breed throughout the world descend from his Beau Monde line. He was the owner of the breed's top producing sire with sixty-five champions and is the breeder of the top producing Bichon bitch.

Formerly a judge of all breeds with the *Federacion Cynologique International,* he has judged championship events many times in Mexico, throughout the United Kingdom, Scandinavia, Europe, Australia, New Zealand, South Africa, the Orient and Central and South America. He has also been licensed by the United Kennel Club to judge most of the 250 breeds that organization registers. In 1995 he became approved by the American Kennel Club to judge all Setters, Golden and Labrador Retrievers, Cocker and English Springer Spaniels.

He includes photography, Central Coast Maritime Museum and Sierra Club activities among his hobbies. A favorite pastime of his is hiking in the Big Sur area with his Boxer, "Raife."

BECKWITH, RICHARD AND LUDELL. The Beckwiths have been associated with Golden Retrievers for more than thirty years. They have produced more than 100 champions and numerous obedience titlists. Goldens of their breeding have been inducted into the Golden Retriever Club of America's registry of Outstanding Sires and Dams, and many more are included in the Hall of Fame. Both Richard and Ludell were professional handlers and now are approved AKC judges. He judges the Sporting and Working Groups. She is approved for all Sporting breeds and part of the Herding Group.

BELL, GEORGE AND SALLY. The Bells' Bel S'mbran Salukis made a considerable impact on the breed and on the public during the 1970s and 1980s. Their most famous dog, Ch. Bel S'mbran Bachrach, was an International, American, Mexican and Venezuelan champion, as well as a Lure Coursing and Field champion. His daughter, Ch. Bel S'mbran Aba Fantasia was also an International champion. She was the Hound Group winner at Westminster in 1982 and the winner of twenty Best in Show awards. She was the only Saluki to be simultaneously number one in both the United States and in Canada.

Both George and Sally, who live in Snohomish, Washington, are licensed AKC judges of several of the Hound breeds.

BELMONT, AUGUST, JR. One of the early fanciers of the Smooth Fox Terrier in America, Belmont was a wealthy financier and sportsman who maintained his Blemton Kennels in Hempstead, New York. He was president of the American Fox Terrier Club from 1886 to 1893 and its vice-president from 1893 to 1896 as well as the chairman of the Jockey Club from 1895 until his death in 1924. His most influential role in dogs was as one of the first presidents of the American Kennel Club. He was elected in 1888, two years after the AKC was founded, and was its guiding force until 1916.

During his tenure the *AKC Gazette* was launched as the official club publication.

BELMONT, AUGUST IV. The grandson of August Belmont Jr. was a devotee of Chesapeake and Labrador Retrievers. He made history with his first Chessie, Bomarc of South Bay, who became a bench and field champion and attained his CD. The dog for which Belmont is best known is the Black

Lab Super Chief. He was, according to his owner, "a once in a lifetime dog, one of the greatest Labrador Retrievers in the history of the sport." He was not only a great field trial dog, but also passed his abilities on to many generations of field trial dogs.

The Belmonts lived on Maryland's Eastern shore, where he spent time training and trialing his dogs with his wife, Louise. He was chairman of Dillon, Read and Company, investment managers, and he became actively involved in AKC affairs, as had his ancestor. Belmont was AKC treasurer and chairman of the board from 1977 to 1979. He was also active in national and local retriever clubs. He died in 1995 at the age of eighty-six.

BENJAMIN, CAROL LEA. No one familiar with Carol Lea Benjamin's work would be surprised to learn that she was taught to walk by the family dog. A professional trainer, she is also an award-winning author and illustrator of eight books on behavior and training, including the best-selling *Mother Knows Best: The Natural Way to Train Your Dog* (New York: Howell Book House, 1980).

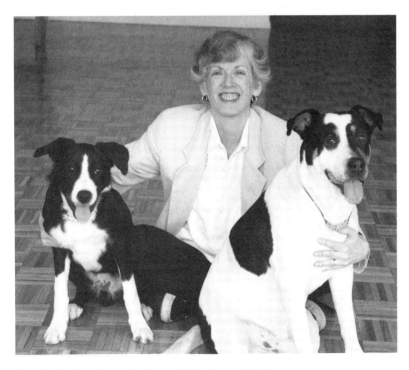

Carol Benjamin, writer and trainer, with Dexter and Flash.

For fifteen years Benjamin wrote a monthly column, "Dog Trainer's Diary," for the *American Kennel Gazette*. She is now writing a dog-related mystery series, beginning with *This Dog For Hire*. She and her husband, Stephen Lennard, live in New York City with two dogs, Dexter, an easygoing random-bred and Flash, a workaholic Border Collie.

BERGER, CHERIE. The Meadowpond prefix is synonymous with Golden Retrievers who are sound, all-around dogs that can excel in conformation and Obedience and still possess the instinct to work in the field. Cherie has raised Goldens since 1968 and has finished many champions and Obedience titlists. Several of her dogs are ranked in the all-time highest scoring dogs list published by the American Kennel Club.

Cherie is an approved judge for Golden and Labrador Retrievers, Irish Setters and English Springer Spaniels.

BERNDT, DR. ROBERT J. Bob Berndt has owned a purebred dog since 1957 and bought his first show dog in 1961 when he started attending dog shows. He has shown dogs in all seven Groups, finishing some thirty dogs and pointing many others while he was actively showing.

During the 1960s he was a member of the Illinois Capitol Kennel Club and has served as a regional vice-president of the American Maltese Association. He has been a member of the board of directors of the American Lhasa Apso Club and a member of the board of directors of the College of Veterinary Medicine of the University of Missouri.

In 1971 Dr. Berndt became a member of the Ozarks Kennel Club, Inc., of Springfield, Missouri, where he has served as president since 1982. He has been the club's delegate since it became a member of the AKC in 1980. He has been a member of the board of directors of the American Kennel Club and served as chairman of that board. He is a member of the Dog Writers' Association of America and has been a member of the Library Committee of the Dog Museum. He has served on the AKC delegates' newsletter, *Perspectives*.

During the 1988–89 academic year he enrolled in a correspondence course on dog judging offered by the Canine Institute of London. He received a certificate with honors at the completion of the course.

Dr. Berndt has been judging since 1970 and is now approved to judge all breeds. He has written nine books, including a book on judging, and during the past twenty-five years he has presented seminars throughout the country on various aspects of purebred dogs.

Dr. Berndt is retired from the faculty of the University of Missouri.

BILLINGS, MICHELE LEATHERS. "Mike" Billings made her debut at the age of seven with a "near Sheltie" at a local pet show. She swept all the honors for best trick dog, best groomed and best-informed owner. Although she may not win awards for tricks now, she has maintained her reputation for best groomed and most informed person on the dog show circuits.

Billings grew up in St. Petersburg, Florida, in a family of dog and horse fanciers. Her father raised English Springers, Foxhounds and Beagles. He was also a sportsman and a hunter.

In 1952 she moved to Stone Mountain, Georgia, where she bred Beagles and German Shepherd Dogs. From 1952 until 1969 her Kings Creek kennel turned out more than sixty champions. One of her Beagles, Ch. Kings Creek Triple Threat, was sold to Marcia Foy, and he made history for the breed both as a show dog and as a sire of forty-seven champions.

In 1962 Billings became a professional handler of all breeds, enjoying a great deal of success until her retirement in 1970. In 1972 she began judging and is now one of seven women all-breed judges in the United States. Michele was the recipient of the Gaines FIDO award for "Woman of the Year" in 1983 and won the *Kennel Review* award for "Judge of the Year" in 1986. She has judged all over the world, including Best in Show at Westminster in 1988. She was inducted into the New York Sports Museum Hall of Fame in 1993.

BIRCH, GLORIA F. Gloria was born on an Iowa farm, where the family raised registered cattle, pigs, chickens and horses. Her first dog was a Newfoundland and later she had a Collie named "Shep." She credits her mother for teaching her how to care for and love animals. From her Dad she learned about training and competition.

When Gloria Birch was thirteen, the family sold the farm and moved to Phoenix, Arizona. While at college there she attended her first dog show where she watched Jack LaRue, a noted professional handler, pilot Ernest Loeb's German Shepherd Dog to Best in Show two days in a row. Then and there she decided to buy a German Shepherd and show it. Her first dog was not a show dog, but she trained him in Obedience.

Subsequently she acquired a good foundation bitch and joined in partnership with Cappy Pottle. Together Covy-Tucker Hill Shepherds have made up more than 200 champions, 45 Register of Merit Sires and Dams, 46 Select German Shepherd Dog Club of America National Titles and 12 different BIS Shepherds. Their most notable achievement was the production of Ch. Covy-Tucker Hill's Manhattan, owned by the late Mrs. Jane Firestone,

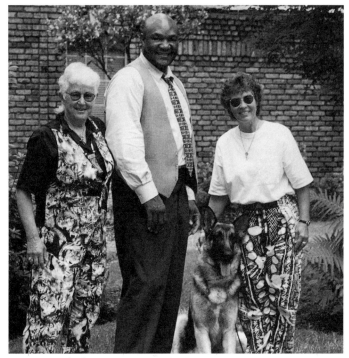

This group includes (from left) Cappy Pottle, former heavyweight champion George Foreman and Gloria Birch with Covy-Tucker Hills Marc Enterprise.

who became the first and (to date) the only German Shepherd to win Best in Show at Westminster (1987).

In addition to her interest in dogs Birch enjoys traveling, playing the clarinet, horseback riding and going to the beach near her home in Cotati, California.

BIVIN, EDD EMBRY. Edd Bivin acquired his first purebred dog, a Pomeranian, in 1952. From this beginning he bred a National Specialty winner. He is the youngest person to enter the ranks of judges, officiating at his first sanctioned match at the age of fourteen. In 1961 he was approved by the AKC to judge Pomeranians, at the age of twenty-one. Since then he has been approved to judge all Toys, Terriers, Non-Sporting, Working and several of the Herding breeds.

With his wife, Irene, he has bred and exhibited Doberman Pinschers, Dachshunds and Pointers for several years.

Bivin attended Texas Christian University, where he earned his BA and MA. He is presently serving as vice-chancellor for administrative services at Texas Christian University.

He has judged in several countries on four continents.

BIVIN, IRENE. Irene Bivin's involvement in purebred dogs spans forty years and started with the training and showing of English Setters. She has also bred and owned Poodles, Dachshunds and Doberman Pinschers. Together with her husband, Edd, she breeds and shows Doberman Pinschers, Pointers and Dachshunds.

Her English Setters were field trained and she has also been active in Obedience, carrying several dogs to their Utility degrees. In 1972 she was employed by the American Kennel Club as the first woman appointed as an executive field representative.

Irene Bivin has been judging since 1965 in the United States and in many countries in South America, Africa and Europe. She has also officiated in Australia and New Zealand.

Edd and Irene Bivin were married in 1978. Mrs. Bivin has two daughters, both of whom are active in purebred dogs and reside in Fort Worth, Texas.

BLAIR, WILLIAM H. Bill Blair joined the Pekingese Club of America in early 1960 and has served as a board member for more than thirty years. During his first ten years in the club he bred and finished more than twenty champions. He became the club's delegate to the AKC in 1970, a position that he still retains. He is also the president of the Pekingese Club of America. Blair is credited with expanding the membership of the national club, establishing a register of merit, adopting a new constitution, code of ethics and breed Standard and introducing the concept of national roving Specialties.

Blair is licensed to judge Pekingese.

BOLTE, DAMARA. Bolte calls herself an "army brat." Her father, the late General Charles L. Bolte, was commander, U.S. Army, Europe, when she graduated from Purdue University with a degree in animal husbandry. She joined her parents in Germany and went on to study sculpture in Paris under Messr. C. Delhommeau.

Damara Bolte was chief of the genetic colony unit in the Scientific Services Branch of the Veterinary Resources Program, a branch of the

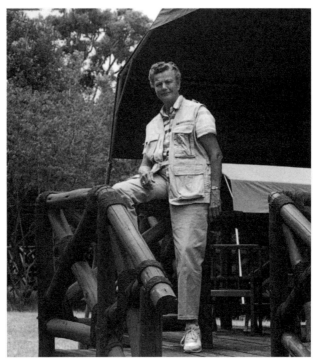

Damara Bolte, professional handler and Basenji breeder, on safari in Kenya, 1996.

National Institutes of Health. She retired in 1992 after thirty-three years of providing and overseeing animal care at the NIH.

Her avocation during all this time was breeding and showing Basenjis, Mastiffs and Border Terriers. Her Basenjis, under the Reveille prefix, made history in the breed, producing generations of top winners and top producers. Several years ago she, with other Basenji breeders, went to Africa and brought back some native stock that has been incorporated into the American gene pool. Her intent was to introduce dogs without the genetic defects that some American Basenjis had developed.

Bolte is an artist who works in bronze and in gold. Her limited edition bronze statues are prized by collectors, and her minisculptured jewelry cast in gold are often commissioned by fanciers who desire accurate replicas of their dogs on pins, earrings, necklaces, tie tacs or belt buckles.

Her main loves, now that she is free of a grueling work schedule, are animals, the outdoors, working with her hands, tennis, swimming and traveling.

BONNEY, FLORA MacDONALD. Mrs. Bonney joined the Dalmatian Club of America in 1913. She was the club's secretary/treasurer for more than fifty years and was its financial supporter in many ways. She often paid the dues of its members and sponsored the National Specialties and sit-down dinners afterward at her Oyster Bay, New York, estate. She took the kennel prefix "Tally Ho" for her Dalmatians; she imported many dogs from England because she believed in outcrossing every few generations. Mrs. Bonney wrote for the *AKC Gazette* and became a judge of Dalmatians, Chow Chows and Poodles. She died in 1967.

BONTECOU, GAYLE. Gayle Bontecou's interest in the Scottish Deerhound started in 1959 when she imported a four-month-old puppy from England. This was the first Scottish Deerhound many people had ever seen. Bontecou showed her more than 100 times, trying to gain a championship, but because they were so rare, it took four years to garner all her points. Bontecou, who uses the prefix "Gayleward," emphasizes conditioning, and all her hounds are worked in all kinds of weather to keep them fit.

Gayle Bontecou, who lives in Clinton Corners, New York, is licensed to judge all Hound breeds and Labrador Retrievers.

BOOTH, KIM. Kim Booth became involved in dogs through his family. His grandfather was Dr. Frank Booth, a well-known, highly respected all-breed judge and breeder of Wire Fox Terriers. His father was Martin Booth, a breeder of Smooth Fox Terriers but more important, the founder of Booth Photography, Inc., in 1969. From the start the focus of the business was to serve the needs of the dog Fancy at dog shows.

Kim was first exposed to dog shows as a youth traveling to judging assignments with his grandfather and by accompanying his father as he photographed dog shows. After serving four years in the U.S. Air Force as an electronic aircraft technician, Kim joined the dog world in 1978 as a photographer. Kim and his father worked together from 1978 to 1985. In 1985, after the loss of his father because of a heart attack, Kim took over Booth Photography, Inc., and has guided its growth into one of the largest dog show photography organizations in the country.

Kim has been involved in Smooth Fox Terriers, Belgian Tervuren, Borzoi and Papillons. Kim's hobbies and interests include photography, dogs, art and travel.

BOSHELL, DR. BURIS. Dr. Boshell, a graduate of Harvard Medical School and a native of Birmingham, Alabama, began his show career shortly after graduation when a patient gave him a Boxer. Although the first dog was not of show quality, Dr. Boshell did his research and bought one that was, a bitch who finished quickly and became a good producer.

Dr. Boshell made his mark as a top breeder with Miniature Pinschers, however, and later as a judge. His Bo-Mar kennels produced more than eighty champions.

Dr. Boshell was a world authority on diabetes and was director of the first public diabetes hospital in America, located at the University of Alabama Medical School.

BOYES, EDDIE. Eddie Boyes is one of the most accomplished handlers of terriers and coated breeds. He became an all-breed licensed handler in 1962 and has made numerous memorable wins, including two Terrier Group firsts at Westminster (1979, 1980) and two Bests in Show at the prestigious Montgomery County Kennel Club all-Terrier show (1982, 1987).

He lives with his wife, Lesley, in northern California, where they manage their large handling clientele and a boarding and grooming kennel.

He enjoys restoring antique autos in his spare time, and he has taken his artistic talents as an expert groomer in another direction. His new hobby is creating bronze sculptures of fine dogs, with many already becoming collector's items.

BOYES, LESLEY. Lesley Boyes came into dogs before she was born. Her mother, Elsie Betts, bred Kerry Blue Terriers under the Tregoad prefix. She became licensed to handle dogs in 1966, primarily showing Terrier, Toy and Non-Sporting breeds.

Her most memorable experience thus far has been to handle the top all-time winning Brussels Griffon, Ch. Wallin's Charlie Brown, to the top Toy dog and Quaker Oats award.

In addition to running their business and traveling to shows with her husband, Eddie, Leslie has raised three sons.

BRAUND, KATHRYN "KITTY". Born in 1920, Kitty grew up with dogs as part of her family's household. A Rat Terrier, German Shepherd Dog and Flat-Coated Retriever were her three childhood canine pets. She first became interested in the world of performance events in the late 1960s when she began obedience training her first Dalmatian. Since that time she has placed more than two dozen Obedience titles on Dalmatians and Portuguese Water Dogs. She has also won championships on as many, including an all-breed Best in Show on one of her Portuguese Water Dogs.

She began a writing career in 1969 and has won many awards for her articles and books. She has written four books, one of which, *The Complete*

Portuguese Water Dog (New York: Howell Book House, 1986), written with Deyanne Miller, won a Best Book award from the Dog Writers' Association of America. Among her greatest honors is the Distinguished Service award sponsored by Fred T. Miller, president of the United Kennel Club, for excellence in communications.

Kitty has been an Obedience instructor for twenty-five years. Much of her career life was as a civilian librarian under contract to the U.S. Air Force.

In addition to her devotion to the dogs, showing in conformation and Obedience and editing the Dog Writers' Association newsletter and the *Courier,* the official magazine of the Portuguese Water Dog Club of America, she enjoys hunting and fishing with her husband.

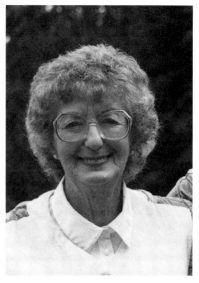

Kathryn Braund, author, editor and breeder of Portuguese Water Dogs.

BREED, MIRIAM. Mrs. Breed was instrumental in the development of the Boxer in the United States. In 1934 she imported a dog from Germany, International Champion Sigurd v Dom, who excelled in the show ring and as a popular sire.

Her Barmere Kennels produced more than fifty champions on both coasts, both in Boxers and later in Brussels Griffons.

BREWSTER, JOY S. Joy Brewster is a noted all-breed professional handler and the owner of Cassio Kennels in Newtown, Connecticut, which she established in 1965. She was named Best Female Handler for 1974 and 1977 and is the recipient of the FIDO award as Handler of the Year, 1979. She has handled top dogs in six of the seven AKC Groups and has shown extensively throughout the United States and Canada.

Besides being a successful dog handler, Brewster has been recognized as an accomplished breeder of German Wirehaired Pointers and Pomeranians under the "Cassio" prefix.

She comes from a dog-oriented family, having bred, owned and showed her first champion when she was seven years old. Both her sister, Sari Brewster Tietjen, and her mother, Mary, have been dog judges. Her sister is a noted writer as well.

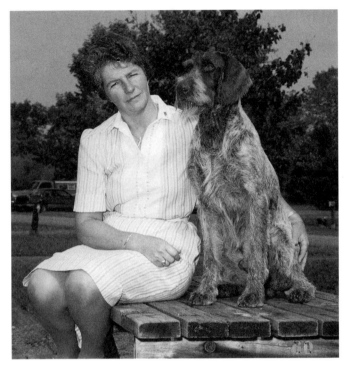

Joy Brewster, professional handler with a German Wirehaired Pointer which she bred, CH. Laurwyn Cassio Mocha Cake, CD.

Joy Brewster apprenticed for eleven years under Anne Rogers Clark until 1965, when she turned professional and established her own kennels. She is a member of the Newtown Kennel Club and the Greenwich Kennel Club, where she has served as president, show chairwoman and board member. She is also a member of the Professional Handlers Association and the American Boarding Kennel Association and is a Certified Professional Handler.

In 1990 Brewster updated her kennel facilities by building a modern boarding, grooming and training building. She conducts year-round training classes and has opened her kennel for canine eye and ear-testing clinics, tattoo clinics, demonstrations and special meeting groups. She works with local schools, offering tours of her facilities and workshop positions for students.

Her most ambitious project currently is to fund and build an indoor-outdoor exposition center that could encompass trade shows, public events and civic events, including dog shows.

BROWN, CURTIS MAITLAND. An honor graduate of the University of California at Berkeley in 1933, Curtis Brown established his own engineering and surveying practice in San Diego. He was a popular lecturer and visiting professor and the author of numerous articles and books, two of which he coauthored with his wife, Thelma, *The Art and Science of Judging Dogs* (1976) and their most famous book, *Dog Locomotion and Gait Analysis* (1986).

Beagles were the Browns' primary breed, and they began their show activities in 1937. They also bred and showed Cocker Spaniels and several other Hound breeds.

Curtis Brown passed away in the early 1990s, but Thelma Brown continues to write occasionally and is listed as a "judge emeritus" in the 1997 AKC Judges' Directory.

BROWN, MARSHA HALL. Marsha won her first children's handling class at Willimantic, Connecticut, in 1949 and has continued in the sport of dogs as a breeder, exhibitor, professional handler, judge, dog writer and educator. With her father, Commodore Thomas W. Hall, Marsha bred, raised and handled fifty Stone Gables English Setters to titles. Named Girl Show Dog Fancier of the Year, 1955, she became Juniors editor for *Popular Dogs* magazine, breed columnist for the *AKC Gazette,* author of *The Junior Showmanship Handbook* (New York: Howell Book House, 1979) and columnist for *Dog News.*

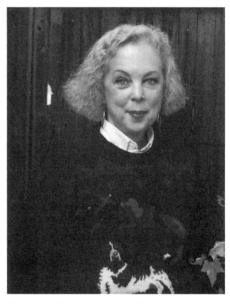

Marsha Hall Brown, judge, writer, advocate for Junior Showmanship.

Marsha has presented seventy-one seminars and lectures in the United States, Canada and Australia, served on the AKC Junior Showmanship Rules Committee, cofounded and chaired the San Francisco Bay Judges Workshop, served on the Education Committee of the Senior Conformation Judges Association, was the English Setter Association of America's vice president and education coordinator and has created the first video instruction for Juniors in the

21

sport. A judge of Sporting dogs, Marsha has also judged the Junior Showmanship finals at the Sydney Royal show.

Marsha has served the Girl Scouts, Boy Scouts and Red Cross and as a graduate of National Aquatic School, was an instructor in swimming, diving, water safety and small craft. A native of Rhode Island, she is married to her high school sweetheart, Robert Scott Brown, has three children and three grandchildren.

Her other interests include museum acquisitions for the Nantucket Historical Association, restoration of her Nantucket home, geneological research and research on women in the American culture. Her upcoming book is a children's biography, *The Ship Rocked Her Cradle.*

Professionally, Marsha is a professor of speech communication in southern California, where she also works as a public speaking consultant.

BROWNELL, JOHN A. A breeder, exhibitor and trainer of Boxers, John Brownell was born in 1905 and died in September 1988. He was a member of the AKC board of directors from 1951 to 1955 and worked on the AKC staff until he retired as vice-president in 1972.

Obedience was his primary interest, and he was approved to judge all Obedience classes and Tracking. He was a member of the Obedience Advisory Committee of 1946 and 1949, and he played a vital role in providing uniform rules for judging Obedience across the country. He performed the same type of work for the Beagle Advisory Committee, where he served as chairman for thirteen years.

John Brownell wrote the first guide for dealing with misconduct at shows and Obedience Trials (*AKC Guide for Dealing with Misconduct at Shows and Obedience Trials*), codifying years of policy that had never been brought together. As he wrote in the guide, it is a question of "whether a family attending its first event would be likely to decide, after witnessing such conduct, that the sport was not for them."

BURROWS, COLIN, B. Vet. Med, PhD, MRCVS. A board-certified internist, Dr. Colin Burrows specializes in canine and feline gastrointestinal, hepatic and pancreatic disease as well as in canine and feline nutrition. His research for several years was to supplement existing knowledge about the causes of gastric dilation volvulus and colitis in dogs. He was named chair of the University of Florida's College of Veterinary Medicine's Department of Small Animal Clinical Sciences in 1996.

BUTCHER, MARJORIE. Pembroke Welsh Corgis in the United States have been influenced since the mid-1940s by the Cote de Neige Kennels of Marjorie Butcher. Before her attention was turned to the little herding dogs, Cote de Neige was associated with many of America's best-known Great Pyrenees. Cote de Neige was located in Bedford, New York, and produced 140 champions since it was first established in 1953.

BUZZARD, JIM. Jim Buzzard has been working and breeding Australian Cattle Dogs for thirty years. He has shown his dogs for about 12 years, producing more than 130 conformation champions, 2 herding champions and several other titled herding dogs.

Ch. Buzzard's Red Tubs HX, was the first dog of any breed to have his herding excellent title. He was trialed four times with four qualifying scores and three consecutive highs-in-trial when he was eleven years old. He is the top producing dog in the breed with more than eighty champions.

Jim breeds dogs that can do everything: showing, serving as companions and working cattle. He has been judging all-breed herding trials since herding became an official AKC performance event.

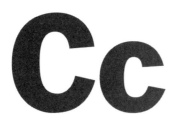

CALKINS, RAY, DVM. Growing up in Iowa, Ray Calkins worked on his uncle's farm during the summer and watched the pheasants and quail develop for the autumn hunting season. His first bird dog and serious companion was a Chow Chow cross! One of his veterinary school classmates bought a German Wirehaired Pointer just before graduation, and when Ray's adopted Pointer was hit by a car in Orange County, California, Ray remembered that fuzzy-faced "hippie" dog in Iowa.

Dr. Calkins's first GWP joined his young family in California, and the red ribbon for a second prize in the puppy stake set the hook very deep! While veterinary medicine at a referral hospital was fantastic, hunting in southern California was not. He purchased a growing practice in Wilsonville, Oregon, in 1976 and began to develop his special interest in canine reproduction. He approaches his profession as a breeder and a veterinarian.

He has bred or owned and trained five German Wirehaired Pointers to nine National Field titles and two dual championships. Dr. Calkins is a member of the Portland Kennel Club and several pointing dog clubs and has judged National Field events for German Shorthaired Pointers, Vizslas and Brittanys.

CAPSTAFF, GENEVIEVE, PhD. Dr. Capstaff was introduced to German Wirehaired Pointers in 1958. She was given Haar Baron's Hans, a dog that became her first dual champion. For the next thirty years she worked closely with Louise Faestel, owner of the Haar Baron Kennels. Upon Louise's death Genevieve Capstaff continued her friend's line.

Her main interest is dogs. She is a charter member of the German Wirehaired Pointer Club of America as well as being an active member of local clubs in Wisconsin and Illinois. She is also active in American Kennel Club hunt tests and dog shows. She continues her interest with a young, promising bitch that she hopes to trial.

Dr. Capstaff is a professor emerita in Humanities. She has remained active in the field as an adjunct professor so that she is able to enjoy the interaction of minds between student and instructor. Her other interests include reading. She loves whodunits, knitting, playing pinochle and continuing research in her field of Renaissance English literature.

CARLSON, CAROL. Carol Carlson's first Soft Coated Wheaten Terrier, Ballymor Heather, was the fifty-first of its breed to be registered in the United States. She has been a member of the Soft Coated Wheaten Terrier Club of America (SCWTCA) since 1965 and is a founding member of the Delaware Valley Soft Coated Wheaten Terrier Club.

She was instrumental in achieving recognition for the breed as a full member of the Terrier Group in 1973.

Carlson has held office as president, treasurer and secretary of the parent club for a total of eleven years and is currently serving as editor of *Benchmarks,* the SCWTCA's national publication. She is currently the delegate to the American Kennel Club from the SCWTCA.

CARMICHAEL, LELAND E., DVM, PhD, Dhc (U. Liege). Dr. Carmichael received his DVM degree from the University of California in 1956 and his PhD from Cornell in 1959. He was awarded an honorary Docteur honoris causa (Dhc) from the University of Liege in 1994 for his work on canine infectious diseases.

He is currently the John M. Olin Professor of Virology in the James A. Baker Institute for Animal Health at Cornell University, where he has served for more than forty years. He is nationally and internationally known for his accomplishments and is the author or coauthor of more than 130 research papers and numerous articles and book chapters. He has received several awards, including two Gaines FIDO awards (1975, 1980), the American Animal Hospital Award of Merit (1981), Ralston Purina Small Animal Research Award (1981), Distinguished Alumni Award, University of California, Davis (1985) and the AVMA-American Kennel Club's Career Achievement Award in Canine Research (1994).

The principal focus of Dr. Carmichael's research has been to solve the practical problems of identifying the causes of canine diseases and the development of means for prevention. His research has also addressed fundamental questions that relate to the way infectious agents, principally viruses, cause disease and the immune response to them, especially in regard to vaccines.

Discoveries that relate to dogs in Dr. Carmichael's laboratory at Baker Institute have included various aspects of canine herpesvirus, infectious canine hepatitis, canine brucellosis and canine parvovirus type-2 (CPV-2). Of particular significance to dog fanciers was the development at Baker of vaccines for CPV-2 and control procedures in kennels, methods for diagnosis of CPV-2, recognition of the modes of transmission, viral persistence and the recognition of genetic changes that have occurred in the parvovirus since its emergence in the dog population around 1976.

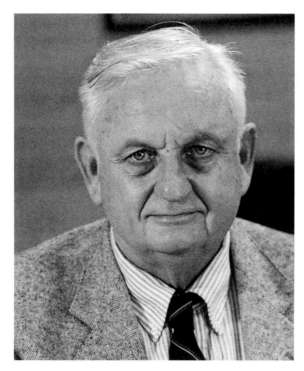

Leland F. Carmichael, DVM, PhD, John M. Olin Professor of
Virology at Baker Institute for Animal Health.

CARSWELL, D. LAWRENCE "LADDIE". Laddie Carswell was a professional handler who started his career in 1938 on Long Island. He was long associated with Spaniels, particularly English Cockers, but it was as a breeder and handler of Welsh Springer Spaniels that he made his mark. He imported his first Welsh Springer in 1961 and subsequently handled the top representatives of the breed to important wins, including Sporting Group placements at Westminster.

Laddie was one of the first members of the Professional Handlers Association and served as its president or its secretary over many years. Laddie's daughter, Candy, followed in her father's footsteps as a professional handler, taking over his kennels and establishing herself as a top handler after his retirement and subsequent death in 1994.

CARVILL, GORDON. Gordon Carvill's involvement with dogs spans forty-five years. In 1951 he and his wife, Jean, purchased an English Springer Spaniel and a Dachshund. Within a few years they decided to concentrate on the hounds and since then have bred and shown more than fifty Dachshunds to their championships.

Carvill has served the dog Fancy in many capacities. He was president of his local kennel club as well as his local Dachshund club and the Dachshund Club of America. He served as show chairman and on the boards of directors of all these.

He judges all Hounds and half the Sporting breeds.

Carvill's main contribution has been as president of the New York State Association of Dog Clubs and the American Dog Owners Association (ADOA) for more than twenty years. He is also president of the Canine Defense Fund, which is administered by ADOA. With its financial help and expert intervention ADOA has been able to influence dog legislation in many municipalities and states throughout the United States.

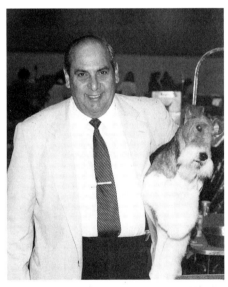

Richard M. "Ric" Chashoudian with Ch. Sylair Special Edition, the top Wire Fox Terrier in the world at thirteen-and-a-half years old.

CHASHOUDIAN, RICHARD. Ric Chashoudian's career in the sport of dogs began in 1944. He has derived his living from dogs since the age of seventeen. During his forty years as a professional dog handler he has handled almost all breeds recognized by the American Kennel Club, achieving top show dog of the year with three different breeds on three different occasions. He was most renowned as a skilled presenter of the terriers.

Chashoudian has won more than 500 Bests in Show at almost every prestigious dog show in the United States, including the Westminster Kennel Club's 100th anniversary show in 1976.

He has been an approved judge since 1983, approved to judge all Sporting, Working and Terrier breeds and half the Non-Sporting Group. He has judged internationally from Canada to South America in the Western Hemisphere, in Sweden, Finland, Italy, Spain and the British Isles, and in Australia, Taiwan and Japan.

He and his wife, Nicole, reside in Baton Rouge, Louisiana, where he breeds and shows Wire Fox Terriers, many of which are offspring of his dog, Ch. Sylair Special Edition (George), now nearly fourteen years old. Chashoudian bought him in England, and he became the top Wire Fox Terrier in the world. He now holds the record as the breed's top sire with eighty-nine champions of record.

After his retirement from the show ring Ric Chashoudian turned his talents to sculpting bronze figurines of show dogs, producing many limited edition works since 1974. In 1989 he added pewter to his line of statues, and recently has begun to produce dogs in painted stoneware. He is a member of the Dog Writers' Association of America, is a prolific commentator and is a feature writer for the *Canine Chronicle*.

CHEAURÉ, ALFRED. A retired U.S. Navy commodore, Al Cheauré became president of the American Kennel Club in December 1996. Mr. Cheauré holds an MBA from Harvard Graduate School of Business, which he attended after graduating from the U.S. Naval Academy. He was a nuclear

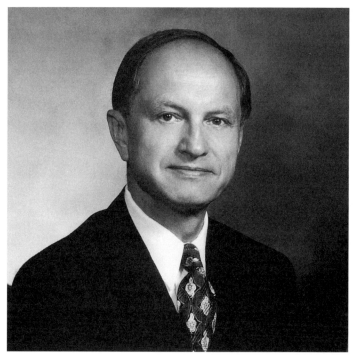

Alfred M. Cheauré, president of the American Kennel Club.

submarine captain and later a deputy commandant at the academy. He retired from the navy in 1988.

He continued to expand his horizons in the business world, working with multimillion dollar corporations before becoming aware of the AKC's presidential search in August 1996.

Al Cheauré entered the dog show world by means of his Golden Retriever, which was shown to its championship. He joined the local Gunpowder Golden Retriever Club in Maryland and became interested in the sport through his contacts there.

On being chosen to lead the American Kennel Club, Cheauré and his wife, Patricia, moved to northern New Jersey. He has been a visible presence at dog events from coast to coast.

CHERRY, ELOISE HELLER. One of the early postwar fanciers and promoters of Chesapeake Bay Retrievers, Eloise Cherry became involved with the breed in 1950 with a dog named Storm Cloud II. She had many loyal supporters, and she, in turn, gave her tireless enthusiasm and energy to all aspects of the sport.

She bred, showed and trialed many of her own dogs, and she held almost every job and every title in the American Chesapeake Club from president to Field Trial judge. She was never afraid of controversy and would fight for those people and ideas that she felt were right for the Chesapeake and for the club that she helped organize.

One of her most enduring contributions to the breed she so loved was her authorship of *The Complete Chesapeake Bay Retriever* (New York: Howell Book House, 1981).

CLARK, ANNE ROGERS. A second generation dog person, Anne Rogers Clark showed dogs that she and her mother, Olga Hone Rogers, bred under the Surrey banner. These were primarily English Cocker Spaniels and the three varieties of Poodles.

Becoming a professional handler in the late 1940s, Anne became the first woman professional handler and only the second of her sex to win Best in Show at the Westminster Kennel Club show. This win was with a white Toy Poodle, Ch. Wilber White Swan. Two more wins at Westminster, both with Poodles, followed in 1959 with the black Miniature, Ch. Fontclair Festoon and in 1961 with the black Toy, Ch. Cappoquin Little Sister.

In 1964 Anne married the late James Edward Clark, and together they bred many noteworthy Standard and Miniature Poodles of this era as well as some top-ranked Norfolk Terriers. Both breeds were shown under both

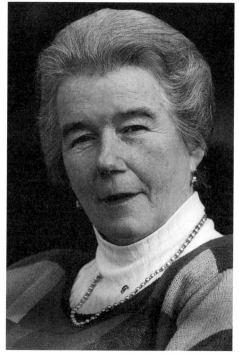

Anne Rogers Clark, all-breed judge, former
professional handler, author and media commentator for the dog sport

their kennel names. Jim's prefix was Rimskittle and was primarily associated with Poodles.

She retired from professional handling after her marriage and became
a judge. In the 1970s she became approved to judge all breeds, one of a
handful of women to achieve this stature. The high point of her career was
the appointment to judge Best in Show at the 1978 Westminster show.

Anne Clark was honored as Judge of the Year and Dog Woman of the
Year on three separate occasions and was the recipient of the first Mark L.
Morris award in 1995. She has been inducted into the Quaker Oats Hall of
Fame.

Together with Andrew Brace of England she wrote and edited
The International Encyclopedia of Dogs (New York: Howell Book House,
1995).

The Clarks have always taken a strong interest in young people. During the time they maintained their kennels Anne and Jim took students

from the United States and from many other countries to apprentice in the handling profession. They taught their students the basics of kennel management, grooming, trimming and handling. Several of their protégés have gone on to become highly successful professionals. Anne Clark judges juniors often and was honored to judge Best International Junior Handler at Crufts in 1995.

She is president of the English Cocker Spaniel Club of America, a twenty-year member of the board of directors of the Poodle Club of America, and she is a frequent participant in breed and judging seminars throughout the United States. She has judged all over the United States and Canada and in many foreign countries.

The Clarks have said, "Everything good in our lives has come from the sport of dogs . . . including our lives together."

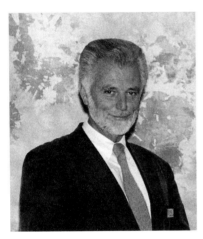

Houston Clark, former professional handler, now a judge and, in his free time, a passionate fisherman.

CLARK, HOUSTON. Houston Clark was reared on a horse farm, and he showed walking and gaited horses until he was in his teens. Shortly after he received his first purebred dog, a German Shepherd, he began training and showing dogs in Obedience. He won several High in Trials and was an instructor for the Chattanooga Obedience Club.

A hobby soon turned into a livelihood, and Clark went from Obedience into conformation. He became an all-breed approved handler in 1964. He and his wife, Toddie, built a boarding, grooming and show kennel, and they handled numerous breeds, tallying a host of multiple Group and Best in Show dogs in all seven Groups. During their careers they won the Quaker Oats Award for Top Dog in their respective Groups four times. In 1985 Houston Clark won the prestigious FIDO award for Dog Handler of the Year.

The Clarks retired to become judges in 1986. He is approved to judge all Sporting, all Working and some of the Herding breeds. The Clarks have been members of the Chattanooga Kennel Club since 1965. They live in a rural golf and lake community in Tennessee, where they are avid fishermen and novice golfers.

31

CLARK, TODDIE. Toddie and husband, Houston, became active in dogs in 1957. Although busy with their four children, Debbie, Jay, Mary and Sharon, Toddie Clark became interested in the dogs when Houston began to show in conformation. She managed the kennel, did the book work and hired and trained the kennel and show help. In 1970, when the children were old enough, she applied for and received her all-breed handler's license.

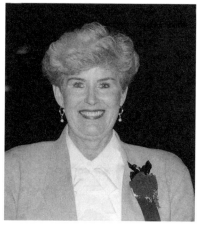

Toddie was a nominee for Best Female Handler. Upon their retirement she became a judge and is approved for all Toy breeds and half the Non-Sporting Group. Today, Toddie and Houston Clark enjoy great demand as judges.

Toddie Clark, former professional handler, now a judge and a partner in husband Houston's love of fishing.

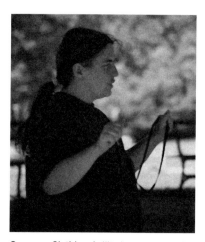

Suzanne Clothier, Agility instructor and breeder of German Shepherd Dogs.

CLOTHIER, SUZANNE. A lifelong animal fanatic, Suzanne is a professional dog trainer with a varied background in dogs that includes breeding, conformation, Obedience, Agility, behavior/training and Search and Rescue. She teaches seminars nationwide on a variety of topics, including behavior, aggression, the athletic dog and training. She is the author of *The Clothier Natural Jumping Method, Agility Training Workbook, Motivational Agility Training,* and *Your Athletic Dog.* The last two are videos. She has written numerous articles for various publications.

Clothier breeds German Shepherd Dogs and shares her life with her husband, John Rice, and with an assortment of dogs and horses. When not busy watching dogs, in order to learn more she can be found reading, cooking, writing, painting and sculpting.

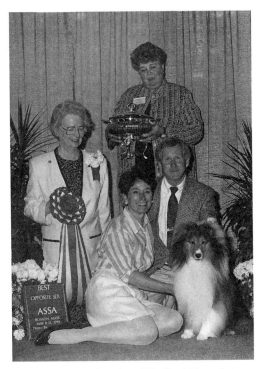

Thomas W. Coen, breeder of Shetland Sheepdogs
and lecturer on creative breeding and breed type
with wife, Nioma, and judge Mildred Nicoll winning
Best of Opposite Sex at the 1995 American
Shetland Sheepdog Association National Specialty.

COEN, THOMAS. Tom Coen and his wife, Nioma, live in the Berkshires and presently maintain about a dozen Shetland Sheepdogs. The foundation for their Macdega Shelties, Ch. Halstor's Peter Pumpkin, ROM, is the breed's top sire with 160 champions. Shelties bred or owned by them have produced more than 450 champions to date.

Coen has served as National Symposium chairman five times, and his interest lies in educational projects. He worked on the original AKC Sheltie video and chaired the American Shetland Sheepdog Association Pictorial Standard Committee. He has traveled throughout the United States, Canada and Japan, presenting his seminar on creative breeding and breed type.

He has been awarded life membership in the ASSA. Among his projects for the future are the adaptation of his seminar into book form and getting judging approval.

COHEN, MERRILL. Merrill has been in the sport of dogs for forty-eight years, judging for more than thirty years throughout the world. He is approved to judge the Toy and Non-Sporting Groups, Junior Showmanship, all Obedience and all Tracking classes.

The breeds he showed both in conformation and Obedience were primarily Yorkshire Terriers and German Shepherd Dogs. He owned one of the first Yorkies ever to win a Utility title and one of the few Champion UDT German Shepherd Dogs. He also owned and showed Doberman Pinschers, Boxers, Alaskan Malamutes and English Springer Spaniels.

Cohen was twice nominated for the *Kennel Review* Owner-Handler of the Year award. He had the all-time top winning Yorkshire Terrier bitch at the time he and his wife, Helen, were showing, and they earned more than twenty-five Obedience and Tracking titles with their dogs. Both Cohens actively participated in both breeding and showing.

Cohen is a graduate of Towson State College (now Towson State University). He taught elementary school before going into business as a manufacturer of medications and water conditioners for exotic and ornamental fish. He is president of Aquariums, Inc., and was on the founding and first board of the National Aquarium in Baltimore.

Merrill Cohen has held many positions in dog clubs. He was president of the Yorkshire Terrier Club of America, president of the Oriole Dog Training Club, vice-president of the Dog Owners' Training Club of Maryland; training director of Canine College; eastern representative for Guide Dogs for the Blind of San Rafael, California; consultant to Southwest Research Institute in San Antonio, Texas, for a government project in the development of the "hand gun dog"; worked extensively with Major L. Wilson Davis on specific armed forces dogs in scent work and Tracking; he developed a program for the Baltimore City Police Department for use of dogs. He is presently a delegate to the American Kennel Club from the Spokane Kennel Club.

COLLIER, CHESTER. Chet Collier is a native of Boston, Massachusetts, and has been involved with purebred dogs since the 1960s. He showed some of the top Bouviers des Flandres over a decade and was an officer and chairman of the board of the American Bouvier des Flandres Club. He has been a member and officer of the Westchester Kennel Club and is a member of its Show Committee. He is a member of the Eastern Dog Club and is president of the Westminster Kennel Club and its delegate to the AKC. He was a member of the AKC's board of directors from 1986 to 1990.

Collier gave up showing dogs in the mid-1970s and became an approved judge of all Working and Herding breeds.

Professionally he is a producer of television shows and has garnered many awards for his productions. He is also in television management and has been a member of the board of trustees of Emerson College, where he holds the honorary degree of Doctor of Humane Letters.

COLLIER, DOROTHY N. Dottie Collier is a native New Yorker, born and raised in New York City. She was introduced to the dog sport in 1965 when she acquired a Maltese. Subsequently she exhibited her first show dog, an Old English Sheepdog. She also showed Doberman Pinschers and later a Pointer.

In 1969 she bought her first Komondor, a breed with which she became identified over the next fifteen years. During this time Mrs. Collier owned or bred twenty-five champions, and she was the owner or breeder of the top winning Komondorok from 1974 to 1984. Her Summithill stock is behind many current show dogs.

Mrs. Collier gave up breeding dogs in 1982 when she became a judge. She is approved for all Working breeds with the highlight of her career being the Best In Show assignment at the 1997 Westminster Kennel Club show.

She has been a member of many dog clubs, including the Komondor Club of America, where she served as president. She is a member of Ladies Dog Club and Tuxedo Park Kennel Club. She is on the board of trustees of Take The Lead, a nonprofit organization dedicated to providing services, support and care for people in the sport who are suffering devastating illnesses.

Dottie Collier and her husband, Chet, reside in northern New Jersey.

CONWAY, THOMAS CARLETON. With perhaps the youngest owner of a registered kennel name, Tom Conway registered Locksley Hall while he was still in middle school in 1947. He began exhibiting Collies the year prior, and in 1948 he imported his first English Toy Spaniel. He bred and exhibited these dogs from 1948 to 1996.

He also bred and exhibited Dachshunds for forty-five years, the last being in 1995, and he bred, exhibited and imported Pembroke Welsh Corgis from 1980 to 1996.

Except for half the Terrier Group, Conway is approved for all breeds, and he has judged in all major areas of the civilized world.

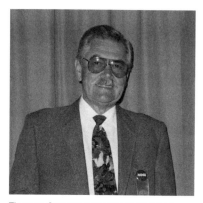

Thomas Conway, breeder of Pembroke Welsh Corgis and many other breeds. Judge of the Sporting, Hound, Working, Toy, Non-Sporting and Herding Groups and part of the Terrier Group.

He served in active duty with the U.S. Marine Corps in Korea during that war. He is a retired educator, founder of Inland Empire Dog Judges Association and a lecturer at the AKC Judges' Institutes. He is a member of the Kennel Club of Beverly Hills. Conway is a writer-columnist for the weekly *Dog News* and a breeder of Scottish Fold cats and Bernberg Trumpeter pigeons. He resides in Riverside, California.

CORRELL, HAROLD. Number one professional handler, the first professional handler approved by the American Kennel Club, Harold Correll was one of the world's foremost authorities on show dogs. He was widely recognized as a consultant, judge, breeder and trainer, and throughout his long career he finished more than 500 champions. His career spanned the years from about 1930 until his death at the age of sixty-seven in 1966.

In 1947 and in 1955 he was honored as Dogdom's Man of the Year. He was a director of the Irish Setter Club of America, a member of the Somerset Hills Kennel Club and of the Professional Handlers' Association. He was a competitor to be reckoned with by his peers, respected for presenting his dogs well, but giving no quarter in the show ring. Business aside, he had a wonderful sense of humor.

COVEY, CAMERON. Cameron Covey is considered to be one of the matriarchs of the American Cocker Spaniel world. She campaigned dogs from the 1940s almost until the present. Her son, Bob Covey, has carried on the tradition in the breed, becoming one of the top handlers of Cockers in the United States today.

COX, HERSCHEL. Herschel Cox bought his first French Bulldog for his wife, Doris, in 1970. Since then they have finished forty-seven Frenchies to their championships. They are the breeders of Ch. Cox's Goodtime Charlie Brown, the top producer of champions of all time with sixty-three champion gets to date. Although well into their seventies, the Cox's still raise and show Frenchies. Herschel Cox was accorded the singular honor of being named to judge the French Bulldog Club of America's Centennial Specialty in 1997.

CROWE, THOMAS. Tom Crowe, chairman of the board of MB-F, Inc., dog show superintendents, has been active in the sport for more than fifty years. He began by buying a Great Dane puppy that he exhibited. He became a professional handler, pursuing that career for fifteen years and then became an approved AKC superintendent. He has been a superintendent for nearly thirty-five years, building his business into a multimillion dollar corporation.

In the early 1960s he began his career as part-owner and superintendent with the Bow Dog Show organization, based in Detroit, Michigan. In 1967 he moved to North Carolina and acquired ownership of Moss Dog shows and the major interest in the Bow organization in 1970. The company became known as Moss-Bow. In 1973 he took over management of

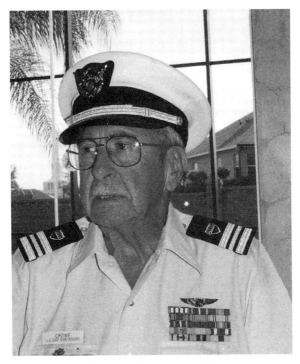

Thomas Crowe, chairman of the board of MB-F, Inc., and an active member of the U.S. Coast Guard Auxiliary.

the Foley Dog Show Organization, and in 1977 the companies were merged to become MB-F, Inc. This organization has grown to be the largest of its kind in the world, directing more than 1,048 approved dog events each year.

As far back as his association with the Bow organization, he introduced the business to the age of computers. He has been a prime innovator of the use of computer technology to take entries, to dispense show and judges' information and to use the new system called InfoDog.

Crowe retired in 1985 from the daily activities of superintending, turning over the day-to-day operations along with 48 percent of the corporate stock to the employees. He now resides in Orlando, Florida, with his wife, Lois, and their Toy Poodle, T. J. Fuzzie. He is still active in the planning and development of better methods of helping participants in the sport. He is still very much interested in computers and is in almost daily contact with the North Carolina office.

Since retirement his other interests center on the activities of the U.S. Coast Guard. He holds the equivalent rank of lieutenant commander as well as aircraft commander and is a member of the national staff of the U.S. Coast Guard Auxiliary as the branch chief of operational flight standards and training. He serves on two quality action teams for the Coast Guard, one in Washington, D.C., and the other in the Seventh Coast Guard District in Miami, Florida.

He has had a pilot's license since 1938, serving in the air corps during World War II. At seventy-nine years of age he plans to give up his active participation in flying but will remain with the Coast Guard in an advisory status. He thrives on activity, saying, "It keeps me young—only seventy-nine going on fifty-four."

His main interests are still dog shows and maintaining the integrity of the sport, the improvement of the quality of shows, the continued advancement of better methods of producing shows plus the promotion and publicizing the joys of owning and showing a purebred dog.

CROWLEY, JAMES. Jim attended Boston College and the New York University Graduate School of Business Administration. He is a former officer in the New York Army National Guard, and prior to joining AKC in 1971 he was with the Wall Street firm of Brown Brothers, Harriman.

At AKC he has held numerous executive positions, primarily in the events area and has served as AKC management liaison to many board and delegate committees. He was the AKC Staff Committee chairman for the 1984 AKC Centennial Show. Since 1993 Crowley has served as AKC secretary. In this capacity he keeps the records of all AKC meetings, has charge

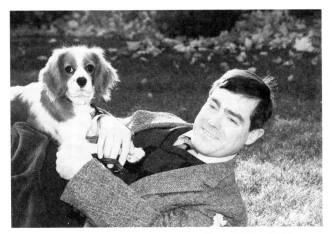

James Crowley, secretary of the American Kennel Club with his Cavalier King Charles Spaniel, Randy.

of all records and papers of the club, is curator of the art collection and is the trial board witness on the show rules. His duties also include the *AKC Gazette,* public and club relations and the library.

He has been a member of the Westbury Kennel Association for more than twenty years and was a member of that club's board before the implementation of AKC rules against its employees holding club offices. He and his wife own a seven-year-old Cavalier King Charles Spaniel named Randy.

Crowley's outside interests include a voracious appetite for reading, college sports and collecting antiques.

CZECH, ARLENE. Papillons have been Arlene Czech's breed since 1954. In 1955 she imported a dog from England to breed to her bitch. Out of this combination she got six champions, including the first Mexican champion in the breed. She takes all her Papillons through Obedience and every champion has at least a CD degree. She had the first UD Papillon, and that dog is still the only one to finish his degree at a Specialty show.

Czech has been judging since 1967, is approved for the Toy and Non-Sporting Groups and several Herding breeds as well as Junior Showmanship and Best in Show.

She is the delegate to AKC from the Papillon Club of America and is its judges' education coordinator. She was instrumental in the production of the PCA's illustrated Standard. She writes for a variety of publications and is also a member of the AKC delegates' Health Committee.

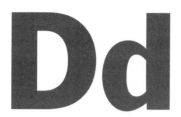

Dd

D'AMBRISI, RICHARD H. Dick D'Ambrisi was AKC's first full-time director of Obedience when he joined the AKC staff in 1972. In his short tenure he made a lasting impression on the sport. Under his guidance the first guide for Obedience judges was started. He was deeply devoted to the sport of Obedience and to purebred dogs and brought his enthusiasm to his work.

Dick lived in New Jersey where he owned and operated a metal fabricating business before he joined the AKC. He was active in all phases of the sport from 1951 when he began in Obedience with a Dalmatian, a Poodle and a German Shorthaired Pointer. He was a member, often a director or officer, of many breed and Obedience clubs, where he also served as training director. He was an approved judge for all Obedience classes and Tracking.

After he died in 1973, a special award was initiated in his name for those who made significant contributions to the sport of Obedience.

DANIELS, JUDITH V. Mrs. Daniels was elected president of the American Kennel Club in March 1995, the first woman to be chosen for that position. She was a breeder and owner-handler of more than thirty Staffordshire Bull Terriers and a founding member of the Staffordshire Bull Terrier Club. She served as an AKC delegate and a board member before her appointment as president.

Before joining the AKC staff she was the chief executive officer and chief financial officer of Daniels Engraving Company, a business she shared with her husband, William. She is a graduate of Kansas State University and holds an MBA from the University of Phoenix.

Mrs. Daniels served as president for one year. Subsequently she started her own vitamin supplements mail-order business.

DEARINGER, JAMES. Jim Dearinger was vice-president of Obedience and Tracking events for the AKC, assuming the position of director vacated by the death of Dick D'Ambrisi in 1973. From 1985 to 1993 he was corporate secretary.

Under Dearinger's leadership the AKC established its first Judges' Seminar in Obedience. He established the requirements for an Obedience Trial Championship, an Advanced Tracking title (TDX) and a Variable Surface

Tracking title (VST). He also established the first National Invitational Obedience Championship, and he was instrumental in the development of the Canine Good Citizen Program.

In 1995 Dearinger was awarded the prestigious FIDO Obedience Award as "one who has contributed significantly to the advancement of obedience training for dogs and to the advancement of the sport of Obedience competition."

Jim Dearinger resides in New York City with his wife, Janet, and their Cairn Terrier, "Lexi." He retired from the AKC in April 1997.

DE LA TORRE BUENO, IRIS. The kennel name by which Miss de la Torre Bueno was recognized worldwide was registered by her mother in 1917 as All Celia's. She bred Brussels Griffons starting in the 1920s for more than sixty years, producing more than 100 champions. She wrote the *AKC Gazette* breed column for several decades and was the president of the American Brussels Griffon Association and an approved judge of all Toy breeds for many years.

DE MUND, JOHN, DR. The seventh president of the American Kennel Club, Dr. de Mund served in that capacity from 1923 to 1932. He was a physician, a Borzoi breeder and a judge. He did a great deal to build the American Kennel Club since he was associated with it in 1909, being one of the original twenty-seven members when the organization was incorporated.

DEL DEO, RALPH N. Ralph Del Deo's activities with purebred dogs commenced in the early 1950s. He and his wife, Blanche, have owned, exhibited and bred Pointers, German Shepherd Dogs, Wirehaired Dachshunds and Wire Fox Terriers. They were successful in producing home-bred champions in Dachshunds, Fox Terriers and Pointers. Their principal interest has been in Pointers, and they have owned and bred many champions, Best in Show, Group and Specialty winners. They bred and owned the last all-breed Best in Show and National Specialty winning Pointer to have won an AKC Field Trial stake.

Del Deo is a past president and honorary life member of both the American Pointer Club and Twin Brooks Kennel Club. He is one of the original members of the Garden State Terrier Club and founder and first president of the New Jersey Federation of Dog Clubs. He has also been a member of the Somerset Hills Kennel Club and Sussex Hills Kennel Club and for more than twenty-five years has served as delegate to the American Kennel Club from the Orange Empire Dog Club. He is also chairman of the AKC Northeastern Trial Board.

41

Del Deo is an approved AKC judge for all Sporting and Hound breeds and has judged in England, Europe and Canada as well as at many of the most prestigious shows in the United States. He has judged the Sporting Group at Westminster and has officiated at many National Specialties for Sporting breeds.

Professionally, Del Deo is a senior partner in a New Jersey law firm and holds degrees from Princeton University and Rutgers Law School. He has written many books on court procedure and evidence and has been a member of the New Jersey Supreme Court Committee on Rules as well as other judicial and legal committees. He is a fellow of the American Bar Foundation and is admitted to practice before the Supreme Court.

He is a former member on the Board of Institutional Trustees of the State of New Jersey and has served on the boards of public corporations and numerous charitable, educational and nonprofit institutions.

Ralph and Blanche Del Deo reside in Bedminster, New Jersey. They have four children and eight grandchildren. They continue to own and exhibit Pointers.

DEPASS, COLONEL M. B. United States Army Retired, of Pass Christian, Mississippi, DePass spent six years as military attaché at Victoria, South Africa. While there, he became interested in Rhodesian Ridgebacks and established the Swahili Kennels. Colonel DePass's Ch. Jeff Davis of Swahili was the first Rhodesian Ridgeback in the United States to finish his championship. Colonel DePass served as the first president of the Rhodesian Ridgeback Club of the United States and was very instrumental in its success. He was very knowledgeable and wrote many helpful articles on the care, treatment and history of the breed while serving as club president and chairman of a health forum.

DESHON, LOUISE. The first Follyhoun Otter Hound came to the DeShons in 1972. He was Am., Can. Ch. Andel Milk Bank, ROM, HOF, winner of five Bests in Show. He proved to be a valuable producer for the Follyhoun line. Because of their occupation, dairy farming in Missouri, the DeShons have had to restrict their show activities and have not raised many litters themselves, though they have cobred a significant number of dogs that became important to the breed. Louise DeShon is breed columnist for the AKC Gazette and is actively involved in the working aspects of the Otter Hound.

DEUBLER, MARY JOSEPHINE, VMD, PhD. The first woman graduate of the School of Veterinary Medicine of the University of Pennsylvania, Dr. Deubler graduated in 1938 and joined the faculty there in 1946. She retired

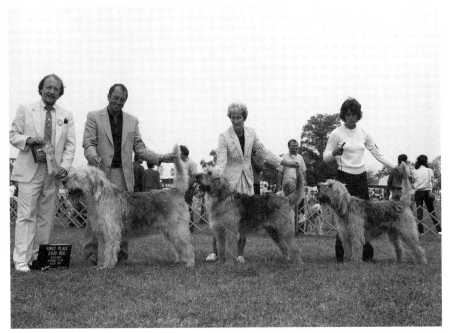

Louise DeShon, longtime breeder of Otter Hounds, shown winning the Stud Dog class at the National Specialty in 1985. The dogs are (from left) Ch. Follyhoun First In Line with Rex DeShon Jr., Ch. Avitar Follyhoun Kahootz with Louise DeShon, Ch. Chaucer's Queen Gwenevere with Jill Battenburg.

as emerita assistant professor of pathology in medicine in 1988 and is presently special assistant to the dean.

Throughout her long, distinguished career Dr. Deubler has built a reputation for integrity, capability, knowledge and the willingness to tackle any job and do it well. She was the organizer of the first seminar for dog fanciers in the country and has chaired this annual event at the Small Animal Hospital at the University of Pennsylvania for twenty-seven years.

In her honor the School of Veterinary Medicine is establishing the Dr. M. Josephine Deubler Laboratory for Medical Genetics, the purpose of which will be to provide diagnostic facilities and training for students in this field.

Dr. Deubler was a breeder of Terriers, primarily Dandie Dinmonts, and she was secretary of the Dandie Dinmont Terrier Club of America for almost eighteen years. She is currently show chairwoman for the American Fox Terrier Club as well as show chairwoman for the Bucks County and Montgomery County Kennel Clubs. She is the AKC delegate from the Bucks

County Kennel Club, a member of the American Veterinary Medical Association, the Bucks-Montgomery Veterinary Medical Association, where she is an officer and the secretary of the Animal Rescue League of Philadelphia. She has written columns for the *AKC Gazette* and for other canine publications.

Dr. Deubler is approved to judge all Hounds and all Terrier breeds.

DICK, ALFRED M. Al Dick was the twelfth president of the American Kennel Club and its first full-time president. He was elected to that post in 1968 and served until his retirement in 1971. Prior to that he was a field representative, executive secretary and executive vice-president. Under his tenure the provisional judging system was introduced as well as the formulation of Obedience regulations and the initial expansion of the field representative system.

Al Dick was a former president of the Kennel Club of Philadelphia and an active member of the Bryn Mawr Kennel Club. He was a Dachshund breeder, exhibitor and judge and served as delegate for several clubs during his involvement with the Fancy.

Before joining the AKC staff Al Dick was an investment banker. He died at the age of eighty-five in 1986.

DOANE, DAVID, MD. Dr. Doane is a retired U.S. Army colonel who met his first dog, a Dalmatian, while he was an intern at the naval academy. Upon graduation and starting his medical career, he bought and showed his first Dalmatian. That began a long line of Green Starr Dalmatians, one of which, Ch. Green Starr's Colonel Joe, became America's top show dog.

Dr. Doane has served the Dalmatian Club of America as a member of the board of directors, president and as delegate to the AKC. He currently serves as chairman of the Dalmatian Club of America Foundation Grant Review Committee.

Dr. Doane and his wife, Marjorie, became de facto historians and archivists for the breed and Marjorie has served on the board of governors and as club secretary. Both Dr. and Mrs. Doane are AKC judges. He judges all Terriers, Toys and Non-Sporting breeds. She judges all Non-Sporting breeds and Toy Poodles.

DODDS, W. JEAN, DVM. Dr. Dodds was born in Shanghai, China, in 1941. She received her DVM in 1964 from the Ontario Veterinary College, and a year later she moved to the New York State Health Department in Albany and began comparative studies of animals with inherited and acquired bleeding diseases. This work continued full time until 1986 when she moved

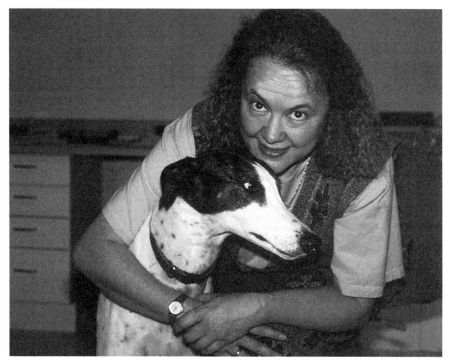

W. Jean Dodds, DVM, hematologist, lecturer, research scientist and founder of Hemopet with one of her rescued Greyhounds.

to southern California to establish Hemopet, the first nonprofit national blood bank for animals.

From 1965 to 1986 she was a member of many national and international committees on hematology, animal models of human disease, veterinary medicine and laboratory animal science. She has published more than 150 research papers. In 1974 Dr. Dodds was selected as Outstanding Woman Veterinarian of the Year by the American Veterinary Medical Association. In 1977 she received the Region I award for Outstanding Service to the Veterinary Profession from the American Animal Hospital Association. In 1984 she was awarded the Centennial Medal from the University of Pennsylvania School of Veterinary Medicine, and in 1987 she was elected a distinguished Practitioner of the National Academy of Practice in Veterinary Medicine. In 1994 she was given the Holistic Veterinarian of the Year Award from the American Holistic Veterinary Medical Association. She was twice the recipient of the Gaines FIDO award for Dogdom's Woman of the Year.

Dr. Dodds is actively expanding Hemopet's range of nonprofit services and educational activities. The animal blood bank program provides canine blood components, blood bank supplies and related services throughout North America. Hemopet's retired Greyhound blood donors are adopted as pets through the Pet Life-Line arm of the project.

Dr. Dodds is a much sought-after consultant in clinical pathology, lecturing throughout the country on hematology, blood banking, immunology, endocrinology, nutrition and holistic medicine. She is also the editor of *Advances in Veterinary Science and Comparative Medicine* for Academic Press.

Her major achievements in research have been the identification of specific inherited bleeding diseases in dogs that are analogous to their human counterparts. Dr. Dodds first described von Willebrand's disease in dogs in 1970, and it is now known to affect more than sixty breeds. She also identified other bleeding disorders and developed readily accessible diagnostic screening processes for breeders to allow them to eliminate carrier dogs from their breeding programs. Current studies are focusing on genetically predisposed diseases that affect canine health with emphasis on thyroid disease. Dr. Dodds is studying the effects of vaccines, drugs, environmental toxins and nutrition on the development and expression of hypothyroidism and immune dysfunction. She resides in Santa Monica, California.

DODGE, GERALDINE ROCKEFELLER. Mrs. Dodge was a famous breeder of Bloodhounds, German Shepherd Dogs and as many as eighty-five different breeds that she maintained at her estate in Madison, New Jersey. Her primary interest, however, was with the English Cocker Spaniel, and she is credited with bringing the English Cocker into its own in the United States. Through her efforts, she was able to persuade the American Kennel Club to recognize the breed in 1946 as separate and distinct from the American Cocker that evolved from it.

Mrs. Dodge was a remarkable woman, blessed with intelligence, exquisite taste, a love of dogs and horses and the wealth to pursue her interests. Giralda Farms, her home in rural Madison, New Jersey, was a showplace, which she opened to the public once a year on the occasion of the Morris & Essex Kennel Club dog show. That show, which was last held in 1957 has never been equaled in elegance or splendor. Every detail bore the stamp of Mrs. Dodge's attention. Trophies were of sterling silver. Butlers in uniform served luncheon under huge tents for the exhibitors and judges. The grounds were impeccable, ringed by specimen trees and flower gardens. By the mid-1950s the show had become so large that Mrs. Dodge felt she could not control it, so it was discontinued. She turned her energies to the establishment of an animal shelter, St. Hubert's Giralda, and set aside an area on her estate for it.

Mrs. Dodge was an inveterate collector of dog and horse art as well as of other genre. After her death in 1973, at age ninety-one, trustees of the estate set aside the best of the canine art collection and disposed of the rest at a series of auctions held at the estate and at Sotheby's in New York City. The proceeds from the canine art went to endow St. Hubert's Giralda, and to build a gallery to house the artwork, bronzes and trophies that remained in the shelter's possession.

DOWNING, MELBOURNE T. L. Melbourne Downing, son of the late all-breed judge Frank Downing, is a native of Baltimore, Maryland. He is believed to be the only second generation all-breed judge in AKC history.

Downing was born into a "doggy" family and grew up with Poodles, German Shepherd Dogs, Pekingese and Pugs. The dogs he first showed were from the family kennel, Holly-Lodge, carrying on the tradition of his father and grandfather before him. Beginning in 1935, he imported some of the top winning Pugs of their time, and they formed the foundation from which the breed has regained its popularity in this country.

Downing was first approved to judge in 1938 and became an all-breed judge in 1969. He has had judging assignments at most major shows in the United States, including Best in Show at Westminster in 1992. The demand for his expertise has taken him to shows in Australia, Canada, South America, Sweden, Denmark, Jamaica, Bermuda and Nassau. He was selected to judge the "Top Dog" in Australia in connection with that country's bicentennial celebration in 1988.

Downing has been both president and show chairman of the Baltimore County and Catonsville Kennel Clubs in Maryland. He founded the Senior Conformation Judges Association and served as its president before resigning, and he served as chairman of the Professional Handlers Certification Board.

An attorney, Downing confines his practice to estate and tax law, while still traveling to judge approximately forty shows per year.

DRAPER, SAMUEL, PhD. Sam Draper acquired his first purebred dog, a Cairn Terrier, in 1935 and has been involved in the sport of dogs ever since. His only intermission was five years of study for his PhD at Columbia University.

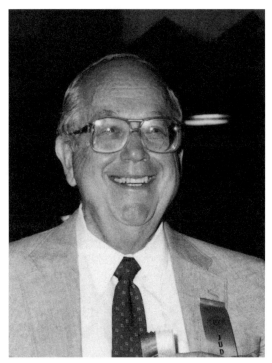

Dr. Samuel Draper, breeder of Chow Chows, judge and
opera devotee.

After that first Cairn came Cocker Spaniels, Labrador Retrievers and
Wire Fox Terriers. In 1963 he acquired his first Chow Chow, Ch. Ah Sid the
Avant-Garde, who won eighteen Group firsts and Best of Breed at the
National Specialty. In 1967, Sam became the co-owner of Ch. Eastward
Liontamer of Elster, one of the leading winners and top producing Chow
Chows in history. In addition to his many all-breed wins, "Louie" won the
National Specialty five times. At about that time Sam formed a partnership
in Liontamer Chow Chows with his longtime friend, veteran dog authority,
Desmond Murphy. Since then they have owned or co-owned six Best in
Show Chow Chows. Sam also was instrumental in reinstating the smooth
coat variety into the breed Standard after it had been omitted since 1941.

With Joan Brearley, Sam coauthored *The Book of the Chow Chow* (TFH
Publications) and a completely new volume *The World of the Chow Chow*
(Neptune City: TFH Publications, 1992).

Dr. Draper founded and directed a mentor-talented student honors
program in liberal arts and sciences at Rockland Community College in

Suffern, New York. This concept has made it possible for students who have achieved an Associates in Arts Honors degree to transfer as full juniors to many prestigious universities throughout the United States.

One of Sam's passions is the opera, both at college, where he sponsors "Youth for Opera," and among fellow dog fanciers. He has organized "Sirius Opera Lovers at Westminster," for visitors and opera devotees who come to New York for the Westminster show. Sam makes the arrangements for the group to attend a performance at the Metropolitan Opera at this time.

He is an approved judge of all Terriers, Toys, Non-Sporting breeds, Labrador Retrievers and Cocker Spaniels. He resides in Monroe, New York.

DRURY, MRS. MAYNARD K. "KITTY". One of the early important breeders of Newfoundlands, Kitty acquired her first dog in 1928, but it was not until she was out of college and married to her husband, Maynard, that she

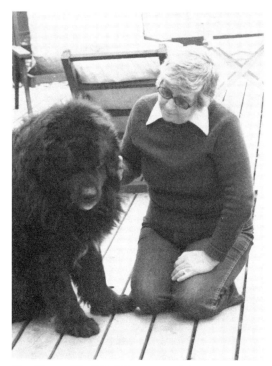

Mrs. Maynard K. "Kitty" Drury, one of the Newfoundland's most celebrated supporters, with special favorite Andy at her home on Upper Saranac Lake in New York State.

began to breed and show in the early 1930s using the Dryad prefix. At one time almost every Newfoundland in the United States could trace its ancestry to a Dryad dog. The Drurys bred about seventy-five litters over forty years. Eventually the Dryad line was taken over by Kitty's daughter, Mary.

Kitty had definite opinions about almost everything, and she would not hesitate to express them. She was a sought-after judge all over the United States and in many European countries. She loved to travel, and when judging shows within driving distance, she usually took a Newf along for company. Her most prestigious assignment was to judge Best In Show at Westminster in 1984.

She was a great supporter of the Dog Museum in its early days and was active in the Newfoundland Club of America.

For many years prior to her sudden death in the 1980s she lived on a lake in the Adirondacks with one or two of her beloved Newfs.

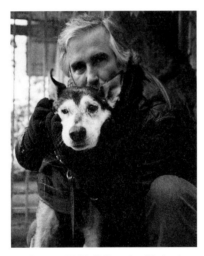

Ian Dunbar, DVM, PhD, animal behaviorist and writer with his dog, Ashby.

DUNBAR, IAN, DVM, PhD. Dr. Dunbar is a veterinarian, animal behaviorist and writer. He received his veterinary degree and a Special Honors degree in physiology from the Royal Veterinary College (London) and a doctorate in animal behavior from the University of California (Berkeley). Dr. Dunbar has three books on dog behavior and training, seventeen booklets on pet behavior problems and eleven videos to his credit. Dr. Dunbar's monthly *AKC Gazette* column on behavior was twice voted best dog column by the Dog Writers' Association of America. He also writes for *Obedience Competitor* and *Dogs Today* in England, where he films his television series, *Dogs With Dunbar*. He is a member of six veterinary associations and the Association of Pet Dog Trainers, which he founded.

Dr. Dunbar grew up on a farm in Hertfordshire and came to the United States to join a research program on dog behavior. He began giving seminars on behavior in 1971, founded Sirius Puppy Training in 1980, started his own publishing company (James and Kenneth, Publishers) in 1985 and then created the Center for Applied Animal Behavior in 1987. Since that time he has given more than 500 full-day seminars and workshops to popularize food lure–reward training techniques. His latest venture is the PuppyDog AllStars K9 Games, an attraction to showcase user-friendly, dog-friendly dog training.

Currently Ian Dunbar lives in California with his son, Jamie, Phoenix the Malamute, a kitty named Mitty and two rats (Socrates and Aristotle). Dr. Dunbar's joys are gardening, sunshine, reading, riding, skiing and generally "hanging out" with his son and the critters. His dream is to live on a ranch and read novels in a rocking chair alongside Bodeen—a mythical ten-year-old Labrador that never dies.

DUNCAN, MRS. DONALD. Mrs. Duncan's Kaydon Kennels of Pembroke Welsh Corgis made a tremendous impact on the breed during its brief period of activity. Mrs. Duncan died in a tragic accident in 1954.

Through her tireless efforts on behalf of the breed, not only as a breeder and exhibitor, but also as secretary of the Pembroke Welsh Corgi Club of America and its breed columnist for the *AKC Gazette,* the breed became popular in the southern and western regions of the United States. Several kennels established in the early 1950s were founded on Kaydon stock, and the phenomenal influence on the breed by the Kaydon import, Ch. Lees Symphony, has rarely been challenged by any modern Pembroke.

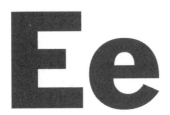

ELDREDGE, E. IRVING. Ted Eldredge is a name synonymous with Irish Setters. His Tirvelda prefix is in the background of every bloodline in the United States today.

Ted considered himself a farmer, and he began his career at an early age in Connecticut, raising pedigreed chickens. He acquired his first Irish Setter at the age of twelve from a respected breeder, Lee Shoen, who thought young Eldredge had promise as a dog breeder.

From that modest beginning Ted bred more than 100 champions at his farm in Virginia, where for many years he also raised a prized herd of Holstein cattle.

Eldredge was a mentor to many breeders who founded their kennels on his stock. He was unfailingly courteous and encouraging to the novice, whether the person's dog was of pet quality or had serious show potential. He judged all setters, having gained his license to judge Irish Setters when he was only twenty-one years old. He judged Best in Show at Westminster in 1980, putting up the magnificent Siberian Husky, Ch. Innisfree's Sierra Cinnar, shown by the youngest handler ever to win that event, twenty-one-year-old Trish Kanzler.

Ted was delegate to the AKC from the Irish Setter Club of America, and he served on the AKC's board of directors, where he was particularly interested in canine health research and education. Ted died in 1982 at the age of sixty.

ELLIOTT, RACHEL PAGE. Rachel Page Elliott has long been one of America's most respected authorities on dog gait. Her unique illustrated lectures have been hailed by audiences all over the world and have done much to awaken breeders to the importance of recognizing the rights and wrongs in the way dogs move.

The book *Dogsteps* (Howell Book House, 1973), was a groundbreaking method of teaching people how to view gait. Based on Mrs. Elliott's lectures, it provided an easily accessible means of looking at dogs. It won the award for Best Dog Book of the Year from the Dog Writers' Association of America. "Pagey" did not stop there, however. She continued her studies of gait at Harvard University's Museum of Comparative Zoology, using the technique of cineradiography to provide fresh insights on bone and joint motion. These videotapes, some of the earliest ever seen, were incorporated into her lectures.

Pagey Elliott, now retired, has lived her life in Massachusetts with her husband and children. Although she owned many breeds over the years, she is most closely associated with Golden Retrievers, which she bred and showed in conformation, Obedience and Field Trials under the Featherquest prefix. She is a past president of the Golden Retriever Club of America and of the Ladies Dog Club (Massachusetts).

EWING, SAMUEL. One of the premier breeders of Irish Wolfhounds in America is Sam Ewing. His Eagle Farm kennel in Pennsylvania has been the home of multiple Best in Show dogs and the foundation stock for many more families in the breed. He bought his first Wolfhound in 1953, and almost every kennel today goes back to an Eagle dog.

Sam is the delegate to the AKC from the Irish Wolfhound Club of America.

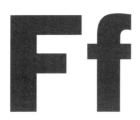

FALKNER, JIM. A boy growing up in central Texas in the 1930s just naturally had a working knowledge of hounds and bird dogs. Jim Falkner was shooting quail as soon as he could stand the kick of a shotgun. The quail were in no danger! He also coursed native jack rabbits with Greyhounds. He started breeding Greyhounds seriously while still in his teens and built up a kennel racing on the major tracks in Florida and Massachusetts. Falkner's wife, Frances, joined him in all his dog-related activities.

When World War II started, Forest Hall, one of the foremost obedience trainers of the day, recruited Falkner for Dogs for Defense. When he entered the service in 1942, he was assigned to the K-9 unit at Fort Robinson, Nebraska, where his commanding officer was Captain Major Godsol. Major Godsol and his wife, Bea, became important breeders and all-breed judges. Falkner spent his entire time in the service as an instructor in the K-9 Corps, working with sentry, attack, scout and mine-detection dogs.

Upon his return to Dallas after the war he began teaching the first Obedience classes in that city. In 1946 the Falkners joined the Texas Kennel Club (TKC) and today are its oldest living members. Between them they have served in every elected office except that of treasurer. They are now TKC honorary members.

Jim Falkner received approval from the AKC to judge all Obedience classes in 1950 and in 1993 became a judge emeritus. He served on several advisory committees from 1960 to 1980 and also assisted Jim Dearinger, vice-president of Obedience events, in a number of seminars on Obedience judging that he conducted throughout the United States. Falkner trained four dogs to their Utility degrees and several to less demanding titles. Two of the UDs were also conformation champions. He served several years as training director for the Dallas Obedience Training Club and is now an honorary member.

Falkner ran dogs in Field Trials for many years and also served as a Field Trial judge. He owned a major circuit champion Pointer.

Jim Falkner quotes an old Irish friend as saying, "I was born a dog man, I am a dog man, and I will be a dog man when they pat me on the chest with a spade."

The Falkners retired to Salado, Texas, where his hobbies are wood carving and painting.

FANCY, DR. GLENN. Dr. Fancy began judging in 1950 and received AKC approval to judge all breeds in 1983. He has officiated at major shows all over the world, including Best in Show at the Melbourne Royal, culminating in the judging of 6,720 exhibits over 12 days of judging.

Glenn Fancy and his wife, Jean, bred Fancway Miniature Schnauzers, which she showed, in addition to breeding and owning Boxers, Beagles, Dachshunds, Bulldogs, Miniature Pinschers, Poodles, Maltese, Yorkshire Terriers, Fox Terriers, Scottish Terriers and Giant Schnauzers.

They have also bred and shown Arabian horses, hunters and jumpers for the show ring and thoroughbreds for the racetrack.

Glenn and Jean Fancy are the only husband and wife all-breed judging team currently approved by the American Kennel Club. Dr. Fancy went to medical school late and received his doctorate in psychiatry at age sixty-five.

FANCY, JEAN. Jean Fancy started judging in 1967 after a successful career of breeding and showing dogs and horses.

She received her basic dog education as caretaker for the famous Barmere Boxer and Brussels Griffon kennel of the late Miriam Breed.

Mrs. Fancy was approved to judge all breeds in 1993, thus becoming the second half of the Fancy judging team. She was nominated Judge of the Year in 1993, has officiated in many foreign countries and was an instructor at the first AKC Institute in Pomona, California. She was ranked as one of the ten most respected judges by the Grassroots Group in 1987.

Jean Fancy raises tropical birds, exotic plants and orchids. She is also involved in interior decorating and antiques. She collects old baskets and American folk art. She shares a collection of dog and horse collectibles with her husband, Glenn, which includes bronzes, prints, door stops, Royal Doulton figurines, as well as a library of research books on dogs and horses.

She loves to attend flea markets, garage sales and auctions in her quest for collectibles. A judging assignment never passes without her finding some treasure to add to her collections.

The Fancys live in San Diego, California.

FANNING, DR. AND MRS. JAMES. Rhodesian Ridgeback breeders from Beverley Farms, Massachusetts, the Fannings established Tawny Ridge Kennels in 1947. The first Rhodesian Ridgebacks the Fannings obtained, Ch. Little John of Swahili and Ch. Moll of Tawny Ridge were acquired from Colonel DePass. Both James and Kay have been active in the Rhodesian Ridgeback Club of the United States, holding positions of president among other offices. Kay continued her activities after James died in 1981 and is still breeding and showing her dogs.

FARRELL, JAMES A. AND EMILIE HILL. In 1934 an Irishman sold two Smooth Fox Terriers to a young American couple who wanted a pair of house pets to bring back in remembrance of their honeymoon. That was the start of Foxden Kennels, which over the ensuing fifty years made a major impact on the dog Fancy through the Farrells' imports and their own breeding programs involving Smooth Fox Terriers, Lakeland Terriers and Greyhounds.

During the 1930s and 1940s Percy Roberts handled the Foxden dogs. Subsequently they were piloted by Peter Green, the Robert Forsyths and, before his retirement, by Mark Threlfall.

In 1966 the Farrells decided to purchase a Lakeland Terrier, and one in particular caught their eye. They bought him immediately but allowed him to stay in his native England until February 1967 so that he could be shown at Crufts. That dog was Ch. Stingray of Derryabah, and he went Best in Show before coming to the United States. The following year he was Best in Show at Westminster under the guidance of Peter Green. Although never maintaining many dogs at their home and kennel in Darien, Connecticut, their dogs made a lasting impression on the breeds in which they were active. Stingray produced multiple Best in Show dogs through several generations.

The Farrells became involved in Greyhounds in 1939 with an English import, and their dogs made important contributions to that breed, as well. The Farrells were active members of the Greyhound Club of America over many years and the GCA National Specialty was held on the grounds at Foxden. James Farrell was the AKC's delegate at the time of his death in 1978.

He was a popular judge, and he was also an avid sailor. He was prominent in the transatlantic shipping industry and was for many years master of Foxhounds of the Ox Ridge Hunt. Emilie Farrell devoted her energies to collecting beautiful artwork, some of which she donated to her various clubs for trophies. After his death, she continued to raise Smooth Fox Terriers, but eventually dispersed the kennel. She died in 1994.

FELDMAN, ALEXANDER. Chairman of the board of directors of AKC from 1972 to 1977, Alexander Feldman was a graduate of Columbia University and received a law degree from the St. Lawrence University Law School. He was admitted to the practice of law in 1932 but did not follow a career as an attorney, instead taking over the family newspaper distributing company on the death of his father.

Mr. Feldman bred and exhibited Great Danes and was long associated with that breed. Prior to his interest in the big dogs he owned Saint Bernards, Cocker Spaniels and Doberman Pinschers. He was active in the Great Dane Club of America and Saw Mill River Kennel Club. He died in March 1983.

FELLTON, HERMAN AND JUDITH. Herman and Judy, who were married for almost sixty-five years, bought their first dog, a Doberman Pinscher in 1935. Thus began the decades of breeding Dobermans, Afghan Hounds and West Highland White Terriers as their principal breeds under the Mandith prefix. They also raised Great Danes, Briards and Dachshunds at their suburban estate outside Atlanta, Georgia.

Both Felltons have been active members of local and national breed clubs. He was the president of the Doberman Pinscher Club of America and for many years served as delegate to the AKC from the Atlanta Kennel Club. Mrs. Fellton established and for years was the spearhead of the extensive Doberman Pinscher Rescue Service, a national enterprise sponsored by the Doberman Pinscher Club of America. Both Felltons were active in local humane organizations and Herman was state chairman for the Morris Animal Foundation.

During World War II, Herman, as an officer in the commissioned corps of the U.S. Public Health Service, was assigned to Atlanta, from Washington, D.C., to establish the headquarters of the Malaria Control in War Areas Command. As the activities and responsibilities of this department expanded, it became the Communicable Disease Center, which today has become the Centers for Disease Control.

In 1953 Herman became owner and CEO of an Atlanta-based environmental management company, which he sold in 1988. He was a registered professional engineer, a diplomate and life member of the American Academy of Environmental Engineers, a Fellow of the American Public Health Association and of the Royal Society of Health. He was a member of the Scientific Research Society of America and the Society of American Military Engineers.

In 1984 the Felltons bought their first Straight Arabian Horse and gradually built their herd to more than thirty purebreds. The horses are maintained on a 300-acre breeding farm, Talaria, located in Newnan, Georgia.

Judy is a graduate of the Arts Students' League in New York and was one of the founders of the Atlanta Arts Festival. The Felltons also achieved a reputation as knowledgeable collectors of Asian art as well as dog art and artifacts acquired during their many trips abroad.

Herman was an AKC-approved judge of all Hound, Working, Terrier, Non-Sporting and Herding breeds as well as Toy Manchester Terriers and Toy Poodles. Judy is approved to judge all Sporting and Hound breeds as well as Doberman Pinschers, Great Danes and German Shepherd Dogs.

Herman was a prolific writer in the canine press, candidly expressing his opinions on the state of the dog Fancy through the media. He died in May 1997.

FERGUSON, WAYNE. A congenial businessman who was once a national brand manager selling Chivas Regal Scotch, Wayne Ferguson saw an opportunity to combine his enjoyment of dog shows and business when he noticed that equipment, vitamins and shampoos were difficult to find. In 1969 he started selling goods at shows and now has several franchised stores throughout the Northeast in addition to his original store in western New Jersey and another in central New Jersey. The big, red-and-white Cherrybrook awning can be found at more than 100 shows throughout the Northeast and mid-Atlantic states and his business has grown to over $10 million a year.

Ferguson is a former breeder and exhibitor of Saint Bernards. In the 1970s and 1980s he showed several of the big dogs to major wins. He no longer breeds or shows but keeps active with many dog-related organizations. He is a board member of Delaware Water Gap Kennel Club and is on the board of St. Hubert's Giralda Animal Welfare and Education Center in Madison, New Jersey. He is a former vice-president of Morris Animal Foundation as well as a member of several community service groups in his area.

FETNER, WILLIAM. Bill Fetner and his wife, Jean, have bred Dalmatians under the Coachman prefix since the late 1940s. Their choice of a breed came naturally because Jean was an accomplished equestrienne, having ridden to world and national saddle horse championships.

Bill Fetner was an air force pilot during World War II and following that tour of duty went into the insurance business, where he became chairman of the board of a large independent agency.

He began judging in 1953 and is approved to judge all AKC Sporting, Hound, Working and Non-Sporting breeds plus Toy Poodles, Collies and Shetland Sheepdogs. He has been active in the Dalmatian Club of America, having served on the board of governors and also as president. The Fetners have considered their dog show activities as a hobby. Their other hobby has been raising exotic birds.

FINCH, KAY. An artist and sculptor from Corona del Mar, Finch acquired her first Afghan Hound in 1940. She also bred Yorkshire Terriers, but her place in history was earned by her owner-breeder-handler success with her Crown Crest Afghans. The dogs with which she made her name were Ch. Taejon of Crown Crest and his son, Ch. Crown Crest Mr. Universe. More than 100 champions carried Crown Crest bloodlines. Finch's career in dogs spanned twenty years, during which time she was awarded a FIDO for Best Owner-Handler of the Year in 1960. She was also a judge of Afghan Hounds. Her bronze studies of the regal breed are still coveted by collectors today.

FISHER, HELEN MILLER. A breeder-owner-handler of German Shepherd Dogs since 1950, Helen Fisher finished eighty German Shepherd champions. She was a professional all-breed handler from 1955 to 1965 and has been judging since she retired from that occupation. She is approved for all AKC Hound, Sporting, Herding, Working and Terrier breeds.

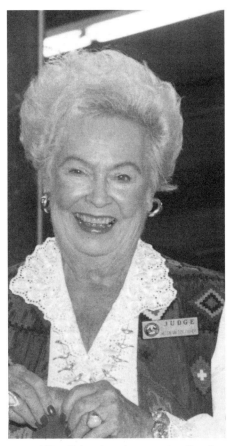

Fisher was the founder and is still active in the German Shepherd Dog Club of Minneapolis-St. Paul, the Minnesota Purebred Dog Breeders Association, St. Paul Dog Training Club and the Minnesota Dog Judges Association.

She has been a board member and membership chairman of the German Shepherd Dog Club of America for thirty years. She was the first and only woman president since its inception in 1913. She served in that capacity from 1985 to 1989. She is presently vice president and national education chairman. She has judged the GSDC National three times, and in 1994 the show was dedicated to her, a

Helen Miller Fisher, breeder-owner-handler of German Shepherd Dogs and a judge of four Groups.

very rare honor. The Wright County, Minnesota, Kennel Club dedicated its two-day show to her in July 1996.

Fisher is active in the all-breed Land O' Lakes Kennel Club. She has a six-year-old granddaughter with the same intense interest in animals that she had at that age. Her hope is that the child will enjoy the same fun and success she has had in her forty-six years in the sport.

FLETCHER, WALTER. The dean of dog writers started his long career writing about dogs when he joined the *New York Times* as a staff member in 1927. He had not started as a canine specialist but was covering all other sports from basketball to yachting at the time he was tapped to report on the Queensboro Kennel Club show held at the old Aqueduct Racetrack in New York. He was to remain at the *Times* for the next fifty years, retiring only because of age.

Fletcher had a weekly column in the *Times* in which he interviewed dog show, Field Trial and Obedience Trial personalities, as well as the rich and famous who were devoted to dogs. He reported on all the shows within the *New York Times* reading area and even went to Chicago and to California to report on the important shows there. Naturally, the *Times* gave him several days of coverage for Westminster. He was even able to cover shows in the more remote areas of the country in his Sunday column.

When the *New York Times* got a new sports section editor in the 1970s, Walter's column was eliminated. The paper received hundreds of calls and letters of protest, but to no avail. The paper has never had another columnist reporting regularly and knowledgeably about purebred dogs.

Walter has continued to write occasionally for other publications, although he rarely attends shows anymore. He lived in the Forest Hills section of Queens, New York, during his entire career. In 1997 at the age of ninety, he moved to Fort Walton Beach, Florida, where he sings in a men's chorus and is taking a drama course.

FOLEY, GEORGE F. Born in 1882 in Philadelphia, George Foley was one of the true pioneers of the sport of dogs. By the time he was sixteen years of age, one of fifteen brothers and sisters, Foley had established his own kennel of Bull Terriers. After 1900 he became interested in the Boston Terrier, then an emerging breed, and at one time he maintained as many as 200 Bostons in his Preston kennels.

As he traveled to shows to compete with his dogs, Foley recognized the need for more business-like management of these events. There were other superintendents, among them Jack Bradshaw, whose organization exists today, but in 1899 Foley superintended his first show. Shortly there-after the AKC licensed superintendents, and George Foley was the first licensee under the new policy.

Foley had the great gift of management. He surrounded himself with efficient people, and he was an innovator. He standardized the services that a superintendent supplies to shows. He attended shows every week-end except for Christmas and New Year's during his long career. He was the founder of *Popular Dogs* magazine, a monthly publication that became one of the most widely distributed magazines in North America. He was instrumental in the formation of the Professional Handlers Association (PHA) and in the conception, with Leonard Brumby, of children's handling classes, later to be known as Junior Showmanship. "The Foley Boys," part of the Foley organization, were responsible for setting up and taking down the show. They were a fixture at every Foley-superintended show and were sought by exhibitors, who came to know them personally over the years, to help load and unload crates, dogs and gear. Even today, the current "Foley Boys," one of George Foley's enduring legacies to the sport, work many northeastern shows, to the delight of many exhibitors. George Foley died in 1970 at his home in Philadelphia.

FORD, FRAN AND JOANN. Together the Fords helped shape the German Shepherd breed as we know it today. Their breeding program has pro-duced many national Specialty winners and established the type known as the "American" German Shepherd Dog.

FORSYTH, JANE. Jane (Kamp) started in dogs as a youngster showing her home-bred Airedale to Best Obedience Dog at a show in Boston fifty-eight years ago. During her teens she managed and handled for Elbac Dober-man Pinschers, Grafmar German Shepherd Dogs and Renfrew and Dorick Boxers. She then became a professional handler in partnership with George Pusey and bred Boxers, becoming the top breeder in the country for three years. Jane's handling career spanned forty years until she retired to start judging in 1981.

Before marrying Bob Forsyth, she, Anne Rogers Clark and Bob worked together at the shows while each had their own kennels. They also en-gaged in lively rivalry in the rings while maintaining great respect and friendship for each other at all other times.

Jane and Bob have one daughter, Sioux Forsyth, also a professional handler. Jane and Bob are the only couple to have both won Bests in Show at Westminster: she in 1970 with the Boxer Ch. Arriba's Prima Donna; he in 1964 with the Whippet Ch. Courtenay Fleetfoot of Pennyworth. Jane was

61

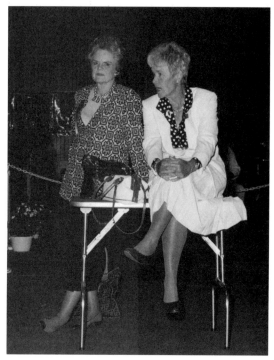

Celebrated former handlers and all-breed judges Jane
Forsyth and Michele Billings (left) "on assignment" in
Long Beach, California, June 1996. "Mike" Billings's
biography appears in an earlier chapter.

awarded the *Kennel Review*'s Handler of the Year three times, which placed
her in the Hall of Fame. She won the Gaines FIDO award twice as a
handler and was once voted Woman of the Year. Jane is approved to judge
all breeds, and she has been an FCI (international dog show organization)
all-rounder since 1981. She has judged in Europe, Australia, Japan, South
America, Puerto Rico, Canada and Mexico.

FORSYTH, ROBERT. Bob Forsyth has spent his entire life in dogs, his
father being a handler before him. In his early years he apprenticed under
Henry Stoecker and Charles Hamilton. He served overseas for three years
in the U.S. Marines during World War II with the First War Dog Platoon.

Upon his return from service he managed Seafern Kennels (Poodles)
and the famed Mardomere Kennels of Whippets and Greyhounds. Forsyth
opened his own kennel in 1949. When he married Jane Kamp, they opened

Grayarlin Kennels in Connecticut and were considered among the top handlers in the country during their long careers. They carried as many as thirty dogs to shows in their big "Blue Bird" converted bus. They were mentors to generations of professional handlers who apprenticed to them.

Jane and Bob are the only couple to have been awarded the Ken-L-Biskit couple of the year. He was awarded the Gaines FIDO for Handler of the Year twice and the *Kennel Review* award once.

They are the authors of *Guide to Successful Dog Showing* (New York: Howell Book House, 1975), which was awarded Best Technical Dog Book by the Dog Writers' Association of America.

Bob Forsyth judges all Sporting, Hound, Working, Terrier, Non-Sporting and Herding Groups, plus Toy Manchester Terriers and Toy Poodles. He has judged in Australia, Japan, Finland, Sweden and several countries in South America as well as in Canada and Mexico.

Since retiring from professional handling the Forsyths have lived in Pinehurst, North Carolina, where they play as much golf as possible.

FOSTER, RACE, DVM. Graduation from a small Michigan High School in 1975 led to enrollment in Michigan State University, where Race Foster majored in physiology. In 1983 he graduated with honors with a Doctor of Veterinary Medicine degree. After graduation he spent seven years as a full-time practitioner of feline and canine medicine and surgery.

His main veterinary interest was the special health problems encountered by those operating kennels and catteries. It was this interest that led him to help develop the Doctors Foster & Smith, Inc., medical supply catalog. Dr. Foster felt there was a lack of medical products and health information available to the general pet owner. Quality products were often restricted to veterinary use only.

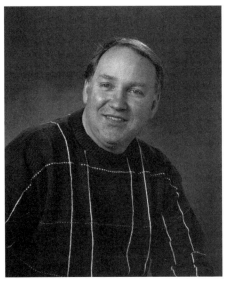

Race Foster, DVM, partner in one of the world's largest veterinary mail-order supply catalog merchandising companies, author and a former practicing veterinarian.

After thirteen years of new product licensing, registration and development, he has significantly helped solve this problem.

Dr. Foster has coauthored texts and newsletters that have been used as educational tools and has also coauthored such well-received books as *What's the Diagnosis* (New York: Howell Book House, 1995) and *Just What the Doctor Ordered* (New York: Howell Book House, 1996) in collaboration with his partner, Dr. Martin Smith.

Race Foster is married to Lynne Larson Foster, and they have four children, including a set of twins. They live in Rhinelander, Wisconsin.

FOY, MARCIA A. Marcia Foy showed her first dog, a Kerry Blue Terrier, at the age of eleven in the suburbs of Chicago. She attended Kemper Hall in Kenosha, Wisconsin, and then Southern Seminary in Buena Vista, Virginia.

She moved to the East Coast in 1961 and began to breed and show Beagles. She had four different multiple–Best in Show dogs, including one of the top Beagles in the history of the breed, Ch. King's Creek Triple Threat, which she bought from Michele Leathers Billings. She bred over eighty-five champions. During the time she was breeding and showing she worked for several handlers, including Jane and Bob Forsyth.

In 1974 Foy combined her household and dogs with that of Anna Katherine Nicholas, and they have been together ever since. In 1976 she moved into judging when she applied to judge Beagles and Dachshunds. She is now approved for all Hound, Working Terrier and Herding breeds, plus English Springer Spaniels, all Setters, Chinese Crested, Pekingese, Chinese Shar Pei, Poodles and Shiba Inu.

Foy is a member of the Connecticut Judges Association and the Central New England Dog Judges Association. She is the coauthor, with Anna Katherine Nicholas, of four breed books, *The Beagle, The Basset Hound, The Dachshund* and *The Fox Terrier.*

She has belonged to many kennel clubs throughout the years. Currently she is active in the Naugatuck Valley Kennel Club in Connecticut, where she has been treasurer and show chairwoman for several years. She lives in Danbury, Connecticut.

FRANK, JAMES. Since 1950 Jim Frank has held an electrical engineering and contracting license. He is a developer of shopping centers and condominium town houses. He is a past president and governor director of the National Electrical Contractors' Association. He is president of the Silver Bay Kennel Club of San Diego, and he has also served for more than twenty-eight years as that club's delegate to the American Kennel Club.

Frank was honored by the AKC in 1996 for his contributions to the Fancy as a delegate and as a judge for more than a quarter century.

He is on the board of directors of the Humane Society and the SPCA of San Diego. He is a thirty-two-degree Mason, Shriner and a member of the El Cajon Elks Lodge.

Frank attended Southern Methodist University and the University of Georgia. He was a navy pilot in World War II with the rank of lieutenant.

He is approved to judge all AKC Sporting, Hound and Non-Sporting breeds, which he has judged for more than thirty years. He resides in El Cajon with his wife, Cathrine, and their yellow Labrador, Cody. He has a daughter and two grandsons.

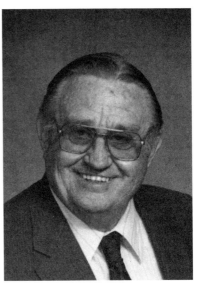

James Frank, judge, president and delegate of Silver Bay Kennel Club of San Diego, California.

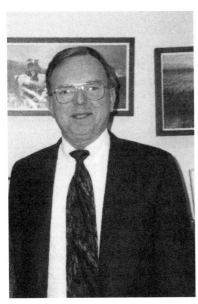

Sean Frawley, president and publisher of Howell Book House.

FRAWLEY, SEAN. An important force in the dog world because of his professional connections, Sean Frawley is the president and publisher of Howell Book House. As chief executive of this highly respected information source on all levels of the dog world, he has made business judgments that have significantly, if quietly, influenced all who learn about dogs from the products of his company.

Frawley started with the company as a consultant to Elsworth Howell, later becoming controller of the company. In this position he guided the venerable organization through a variety of economic waters and always made it to a safe harbor with the help of his keen sense of business acumen. Upon Howell's retirement from active participation, Frawley was named president and became involved in all aspects of the company's operations. Throughout its history and until then, Howell Book House had remained a private company. After Elsworth Howell's sudden death and his family's decision to sell the company, Frawley remained at the helm while the publishing house went through two fateful ownership changes.

Happily, Sean Frawley has maintained his position at Howell in the face of these corporate shifts, and with his leadership the company has not only thrived, but also experienced unprecedented growth. Today Howell Book House offers fine books for all levels of the dog-interested and takes an important share of the credit for the establishment of an informed, intelligent Fancy.

Frawley has actively championed Howell Book House's active participation in many areas of the dog Fancy. The support given to the Dog Writers' Association of America and to the Dog Fanciers' Club are two examples of the president's vision.

Born on a working farm in the beautiful County Clare in Western Ireland, Frawley came to the United States as a young man, served in the military and married a hometown "colleen." Fran and Sean Frawley have two sons, Sean and David, and a daughter, Mary, who presented them with their first grandchild in June 1997. As a boy, Frawley knew working stock dogs well. Today, however, the Frawleys share their Croton, New York, home with "Bailey," a chocolate Labrador Retriever.

FREEMAN, MURIEL. Known as "the Rottweiler's Best Friend," Mrs. Freeman is widely recognized as the leading Rottweiler expert in the United States. She was a founder of the American Rottweiler Club and shepherded it through the processes of becoming the Parent Club for the breed. She served as the club's first AKC delegate.

Muriel Freeman was the first breeder to recognize and take action about hip dysplasia as a leading cause of lameness in Rottweilers. She spearheaded efforts to require radiographic screening as a method of controlling this genetic disorder.

Freeman, a native of Long Island, has always lived in the New York area. Horses and dogs were an integral part of her childhood. She first rode a pony when she was three and competed in horsemanship events throughout her teens. The family always owned large dog breeds as pets.

After her graduation in 1937 from Wilson College in Chambersburg, Pennsylvania, she married Bernard Freeman. The couple raised two sons with a Shepherd mix and two Great Danes. Mrs. Freeman enjoyed golf and became the number one player on the Women's Metropolitan Golf Association team. She made the *Guiness Book of World Records* when, two days in a row, at two different California golf courses, she made holes-in-one.

It was her husband who wanted a Rottweiler, and in 1957 Mrs. Freeman consented to purchase one to please him. That dog changed her life and made her an ardent advocate of the breed.

When she became president of the Colonial Rottweiler Club, a regional Pennsylvania club, the board established a code of ethics requiring club members to have their dogs OFA certified. She considers that to be her most significant contribution to the welfare of the breed.

Muriel Freeman organized the Colonial Rottweiler Club Rescue League and the first Rottweiler Puppy Sweepstakes. She was president of Westbury Kennel Association from 1973 to 1978 and was a board member of the Long Island Kennel Club for decades. She is still an honorary member of that club plus ten Rottweiler clubs in the United States and abroad. She was the first American invited by the German Rottweiler organization to apprentice to judge the breed in that country.

She organized the first Rottweiler educational symposium in Toronto, Ontario, in 1976. Since then she has conducted seminars on five continents and throughout the United States. She was an approved judge for twenty-seven years, although she retired in 1994. She judged Best in Show at Westminster in 1989. She is the author of *The Complete Rottweiler* (New York: Howell Book House, 1983).

Mrs. Freeman's mission has been to educate breeders and prospective owners about the responsibilities of breeding, selling and owning such a large, impressive dog. She stresses to everyone who seeks her advice that this is not a breed to be taken lightly. Although she no longer breeds or shows dogs, her counsel is sought by anyone truly interested in learning about the Rottweiler.

FREI, DAVID. David Frei's involvement in the dog world begins, but does not end, as co-owner with his wife, Sandy, of Stormhill Kennels, one of the top Afghan Hound kennels in the world.

Since 1990 he has provided the colorful commentary for the television coverage of the Westminster Kennel Club show broadcasted each February from Madison Square Garden.

Frei is a past president and current board member of the Afghan Hound Club of America. He chaired the widely acclaimed Afghan Hound World Congress in San Diego, attended by more than 500 fanciers from 23 different countries.

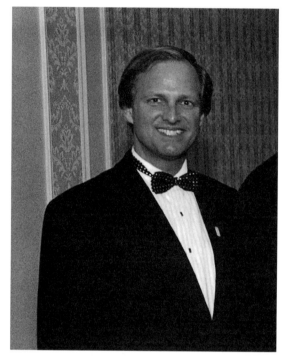

David Frei, Afghan Hound breeder and "The Voice of Westminster" to the national television audience.

Approved by the AKC to judge Afghans, Frei has officiated at Specialty and all-breed shows throughout the United States. He judged the Australian National Specialty and events in Europe and Canada.

Through the years, Stormhill has produced nearly 100 American and international champions, including Ch. Stormhill's Who's Zoomin' Who, the number one Afghan in the United States in 1989 and retired as the top winning female in the history of the breed.

Frei is a trustee for Take The Lead, a national, nonprofit foundation providing support for members of the dog show family suffering from terminal disease or life-threatening illness. He is a member of the King County Animal Control Citizens Advisory Committee and is a past director of the Humane Society of Seattle-King County and for Morris Animal Foundation.

As director of promotions for the Denver Broncos he created and implemented the "Orange Crush" promotion when the Broncos made their first trip to the Super Bowl following the 1977 season. He has also held public relations positions with the San Francisco Forty-niners and *ABC-TV Sports* in New York.

Dave Frei has owned and operated two unique and popular sports bar restaurants in the Seattle area.

He and Sandy live in Woodinville, Washington.

Gg

GARDINER, VIRGINIA PERRY. Virginia Perry Gardiner has lived all her life in rural Rhode Island. She maintains a studio in her home where she sculpts in bronze and pewter and creates breed-specific jewelry in silver and gold. Many of her pieces are limited editions and are coveted by fanciers who look for the latest "Virginia" statue, ring, bracelet or pendant. She does commissioned work, often incorporating diamonds and other precious stones into the designs.

As a child she sculpted animals as a way of expressing herself. In high school she won a national sculpture award and after graduation attended the Hartford, Connecticut Art School.

Gardiner then pursued a career as a commercial sculptor for Hasbro, the large toy manufacturer. This occupied so much of her time that she did not return to animal sculpting until she bought a Great Dane puppy. The puppy was nominated for a Futurity, and Gardiner was bitten by the dog-show bug. Her involvement with dog shows led to the first commissioned pieces, and as demand for her work increased, she abandoned the commercial art world to dedicate herself to animal sculpting. In 1976 she produced her first line of dog sculptures in bronze and pewter.

A turning point in Gardiner's career came when she met Ana Goulet, who became her business partner. Goulet manages and runs the business that has become the A. Goulet–V. Gardiner Studio, featuring the Virginia Perry Gardiner Collection. When Goulet joined the business, Gardiner added a line of custom jewelry in 14K and 18K gold. She now sculpts more than fifty breeds.

Gardiner's artwork is recognized for its anatomical accuracy, expression of character and aesthetic appeal. Her jewelry has won several ribbons at the "Art Show at the Dog Show," sponsored annually by the Wichita Kennel Club. Her creations have found patrons in private collections in Thailand, Japan, Australia, Europe, South America, Africa, most of the Canadian provinces and in all fifty U.S. states.

Virginia Perry Gardiner exhibits at selected shows throughout the year, including some National Specialties and a few of the larger all-breed shows, including Westminster. She can be found by the crowd six deep in front of her small booth, where the business becomes a family enterprise, with her two sons, Chris and Matt, pitching in to help.

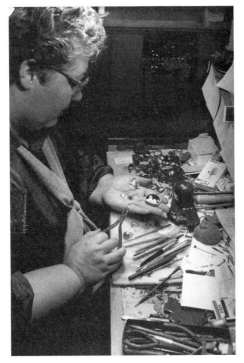

Virginia Perry Gardiner, sculptor and jewelry
designer, in her workshop.

GASOW, JULIA. There are few people in the world of purebred dogs about
whom it can be said that they changed their breed. Julia Gasow is one.
There is no doubt that her breeding program, which started in 1936 and
continues today, put an indelible stamp on the English Springer Spaniel in
the United States.

Julia Gasow was born in 1904 and was raised in Kansas City, Missouri.
When she grew up she moved to the Detroit area where she met a veterinarian who became her husband, supporter and best friend. They raised
two daughters, Sally and Linda, for whom Salilyn Kennels was named.
Fred Gasow died in 1993.

Of the several hundred Salilyn Springers produced over the decades,
none was more influential in setting type in the breed than Ch. Salilyn's
Aristocrat. "Risto" was a top winner, handled by Dick Cooper throughout
his career. He won more than 60 Bests in Show, more than 100 Sporting
Groups and 5 Specialties. This record was remarkable for the time. His
legacy endured through his progeny. He sired 188 champions, including

Ch. Salilyn's Condor (Robert) who won Best in Show at Westminster in 1993, piloted by Mark Threlfall. This was a culmination of the years of striving to produce the perfect dog. Mrs. Gasow got pretty close.

Julia Gasow was the driving force behind the success of the Detroit Kennel Club, one of the few remaining benched shows in the United States. At her insistence, education for the spectators became a hallmark of the show. She felt it essential that the public understand and appreciate the value and the responsibility of owning a purebred dog. Through her efforts and those of her coworkers in the club, the Detroit show became an annual fixture, attracting more than 40,000 people to the Motor City's Cobo Hall each year.

She was the recipient of many awards through her lifetime, including the Lifetime Achievement Award from the Quaker Oats Company.

At the age of ninety-two Julia Gasow is still trying to breed the perfect dog. Her love and dedication to the breed is just as intense as it was when she began as a young girl with a prophetically named bitch, Hibank Hopeful.

GAUSS, CATHERINE DAVIS. Catherine Gauss was one of the early breeders and one of the most influential supporters of Papillons in the United States. She was born in 1904 and was involved with the breed most of her adult life. She joined the Papillon Club of America in 1949, and when the membership dropped away and the club was in danger of dissolving, Mrs. Gauss took over as president and brought the club back together.

She was instrumental in reviving the Standard for the breed on two occasions, and she was the author of *How to Raise and Train a Papillon* (Jersey City: TFH Publications, 1964). She was a great benefactor of the Dog Museum and of the National Specialties. She was the Papillon Club of America's delegate to the AKC from 1979 to 1986.

Her kennel name, Cadaga, was prominent in many pedigrees, and she also imported several dogs to complement her breeding program and to make them available to other breeders. Cadaga entries won the National Specialties nine times, the last in 1974.

GIBSON-SMITH, NORMA. Born in Saline, Michigan, in 1962, Norma Gibson-Smith attended Eastern Michigan University but decided that dogs would be her life. She founded Amron Kennels in 1973 and is a breeder of Bouvier des Flandres and French Bulldogs. She has handled dogs to top wins at National Specialties in both breeds.

In 1984 Smith began her career as a professional all-breed handler, and she has won more than sixty Bests in Show and has made several of her

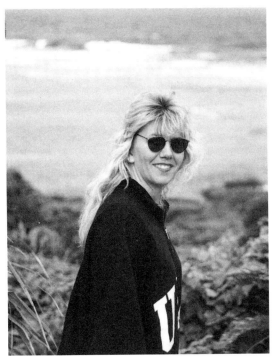

Norma Gibson-Smith, professional handler and outdoors enthusiast.

clients' dogs top in their breeds. She was voted Best New Female Handler in 1990.

Her hobbies include bodybuilding and working out. She has been a vegetarian for more than five years.

In 1996 she married Ron Smith, and she still lives in her hometown of Saline.

GILBERT, EDWARD M., JR. Ed Gilbert is a judge, writer and man of many interests regarding purebred dogs. He is the author of two books and many articles in the dog press. He is a member of the Dog Writers' Association of America, which awarded his coauthored book, *The Complete Afghan Hound* (New York: Howell Book House, 1988, 1975) an honorable mention for best book of the year.

Gilbert is a delegate to the AKC from Channel Cities Kennel Club, where he serves on the delegates' newsletter, *Perspectives,* and on the delegates Health Committee.

73

He has long been involved in the politics of canine legislation on local, state and national levels and in 1994 and 1995 served as president of the California Federation of Dog Clubs. He has also held offices in Orange Empire Dog Club, Afghan Hound Club of America, American Saluki Association, various regional Specialty clubs, Senior Conformation Judges Association, American Dog Show Judges Association, California Coalition of Animal Owners and American Dog Owners Association.

He has been featured speaker at many canine symposiums, and he is a founder of the Los Angeles Dog Judges Educational Association.

During World War II Gilbert served as an electronic technician in the U.S. Navy. After his discharge he attended the Milwaukee School of Engineering and upon graduation went to work for Convair (later General Dynamics) on air defense guided missiles in San Diego. His career included engineering management for several types of missiles for the armed forces, and he worked with foreign navies developing their missile programs. He retired as senior project engineer after forty years in June 1991.

While at General Dynamics Ed Gilbert taught electronics part-time at Mt. San Antonio College, Chaffey College and California Polytechnic College in Pomona.

Gilbert began his judging career in 1969 and is approved to judge all Sporting and Hound breeds, Akitas, Doberman Pinschers and the Miscellaneous class. He has judged throughout the United States and in Australia, Canada, Finland, Israel and New Zealand, where he also conducted educational programs. He has also judged in Hong Kong and in Taiwan.

GLICKMAN, LAWRENCE T., VMD, PhD. Larry Glickman is a professor of epidemiology and environmental medicine at Purdue University School of Veterinary Medicine. He has been a pioneer in the application of epidemiology to the study of pet dogs. This approach is a humane alternative to laboratory experiments for studying the cause of diseases and their treatment.

His contributions in this field include demonstrating that certain breeds are more susceptible to parvovirus infection; finding that exposure to asbestos and insecticides increases the risk of lung and bladder cancer, respectively, in dogs; showing that certain diets are associated with increased survival following mastectomy in dogs with breast cancer; characterizing the dog overpopulation in the United States and identifying why owners relinquish dogs to shelters; better defining the human-dog bond and its implications for the health and welfare of both species; conducting the largest prospective study of pet dogs (more than 2,000) to identify the risk factor for bloat; elucidating the relationship between overvaccination and the development of autoimmune disease; and establishing the first "Animal Welfare and Societal Issues Curriculum" for undergraduate students as a major.

Dr. Glickman graduated from the State University of New York at Binghampton with a major in biology in 1964. He is a 1972 graduate in veterinary medicine from the University of Pennsylvania, and he received his doctorate in epidemiology from the University of Pittsburgh in 1977. Before joining the faculty at Purdue, he was associated with Cornell and the University of Pennsylvania.

His hobbies are golf, gardening, travel and exchanging views and ideas with dog breeders and owners. He and his wife, Nina, work together on several of his projects at Purdue.

GODSOL, BEATRICE HOPKINS. Bea Godsol has been remembered throughout the years since her death as one of history's great "dog people," mentors and judges. She and her husband, Colonel Major Godsol, raised German Shepherds, Newfoundlands, Sealyham Terriers and Beagles at their home in California.

She had a keen eye for a good dog, finding those whom others might overlook. In 1957 she gave Best in Show at Westminster to an up-and-coming, owner-handled home-bred Afghan Hound, Ch. Shirkhan of Grandeur. The dog went on to enjoy a successful show career, but his influence as a producer is still strong today. She launched the careers of many other famous show dogs of the day, but she was valued most by her peers as a friend, advisor and teacher. Both she and Major were pioneers in obedience training, which they conducted at their ranch. They both were all-rounders and judged all over the world for twenty-five years.

She loved the islands and spent as much time as possible in Hawaii, and she was also a collector of books and antiques, which crammed their homes, first in northern California and later in Palm Springs. Major Godsol died in 1970. Bea passed away in 1978.

GOODMAN, WALTER F. A member of the board of directors of the AKC, Walter Goodman is serving his third term in that elected office.

As a breeder-owner-handler of Skye Terriers since 1940, Goodman has finished thirty-five champions he has owned with his mother, Mrs. Adele Goodman. They bought their first Skye in 1935, but it was not until 1947, the year Goodman graduated from Yale, that they had their first champion.

Glamoor Kennels produced many top winning dogs, perhaps the most famous being a home-bred, Ch. Glamoor Good News, who won Best in Show at Westminster in 1969 with Goodman handling her. She is the only Skye Terrier to ever win the top award at this show.

Goodman began to judge in 1977 and is approved for all Terrier breeds and Toy Manchester Terriers. His judging credits include many of America's most prestigious shows. He made the Best in Show selection at Westminster in 1994.

He has been a member of the Skye Terrier Club of America since 1951 and its delegate since 1976. He has been a member of several board committees during his tenure, and he also serves on the board of the Dog Museum and the board of overseers at the University of Pennsylvania's veterinary school.

Walter Goodman served in the U.S. Army in Europe as an NCO from 1943 to 1947. He was employed as a trust officer and assistant vice-president at Chase Manhattan Bank, as an associate producer for NBC-TV and for Mike Ellis Broadway Productions. While retired from his position as president and senior partner of Goodman Flanders, Inc., a contract and residential furniture accessory company, he is still active in this business as a consultant.

Goodman is a resident of Miami, Florida.

GREEN, PETER J. Peter Green started in dogs at age ten in his hometown of Neath, Wales. His uncle had a large kennel of Welsh and Wire Fox Terriers through which he learned how to trim and to show. His uncle was Harol Snow of Felstead Kennels, which is the world's most famous name in Welsh Terriers. His cousin Emlyn still keeps the largest kennels of Welsh Terriers in the world.

After two years of national service in the Royal Air Force, Green showed dogs professionally in England and between 1960 and 1963 was very successful with Welsh Terriers.

In 1963 Green moved his family from Wales, first to California and then to Pennsylvania, where he worked for Mr. and Mrs. William Wimer III at their Pool Forge Kennels. In 1967 he went out on his own and became an all-breed professional handler specializing in Terriers.

The first dog he imported was purchased by Mr. and Mrs. James Farrell, the Lakeland Terrier Ch. Stingray of Derryabah, who won Best in Show at Crufts in England in 1967 and in the subsequent year took top honors at Westminster. Peter won Westminster on two other occasions: in 1977 with the Sealyham Terrier Ch. Dersade Bobby's Girl; and in 1994 with the Norwich Terrier, Ch. Chidley Willum the Conqueror, the first of the breed to do so.

He has won Best in Show at the Montgomery County Kennel Club all-Terrier show seven times since first attending in 1964, and he has won Best in Show at every major dog show in the United States at least once.

Five of his clients' dogs have become winners of the Top Show Dog of the Year. He is a three-time winner of the *Kennel Review* award for Top Male Handler, and he has twice won the Gaines FIDO for Top Handler of the Year.

Green and wife, Gaynor, have four children. Andrew is now a professional dog handler, working with his father. Although Peter is renowned in Terrier circles, he also handles top dogs in the other six Groups.

Peter Green's life is centered around dogs, and he also judges outside the United States. He has judged in the British Isles, the Scandinavian countries, Italy, Germany, Belgium, Colombia and Australia. He often goes abroad to seek top dogs to import for his clients. Green lives in Bowansville, Pennsylvania.

GREGORY, JOSEPH E. Joe Gregory entered the dog show world when he was still in college. He bought his first Boxer for his mother and became a professional handler apprenticed to the great Phil Marsh, who later became an all-breed judge. In 1952 Gregory got his handlers' license. He stayed in the profession until he married Mamie Reynolds in 1966. In 1967 he became an AKC judge and is now approved to judge all breeds. He is a life member of the American Boxer Club, an honor that he received in 1983.

Mamie Gregory also came from a doggy family. Her family raised Doberman Pinschers, and her first dog was a Cocker Spaniel that she took into the show ring when she was eight years old. This was the first of a long line of winning show dogs for her and eventually for both of them. Their greatest success came with a Maltese, Ch. Joanne-Chen's Maya Dancer, who won more than 100 Groups and was a two-time winner of the Ken-L-Ration award for Top Toy dog.

GRIVAS, DENIS. Another Welshman and another of the rare club of all-rounders, Denis Grivas has been in dogs all his life. His whole family in Wales bred and owned Terriers—Scotties and Fox Terriers—Smooth and Wire. When he emigrated to the United States before World War II, he began to breed and show Boxers, which he bred for thirty-five years. He began to handle professionally in 1952 and in 1963 decided to become a judge. He has lived in New Orleans, Louisiana, since he arrived on these shores.

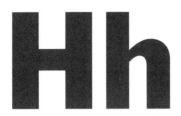

Hh

HAGGERTY, CAPTAIN ARTHUR. Captain Haggerty is a leader in the field of dog training and instruction. He has trained with and supplied security, bomb and drug dogs to such diverse organizations as the Panamanian Defense Force and Macy's. He has also trained dogs for the London, England metropolitan police, Scotland Yard and the Berlin, Germany Police Department. He is a former training officer for the U.S. Army and Air Force, and he has trained dogs for the Palm Beach County Sheriff's Department.

During the 1960s and 1970s he worked with Duke University's parapsychology laboratory, and he established the National Dog Bite Fatality Investigation Committee. He worked with scientists in Germany analyzing the dog's olfactory acuity, and he was civilian consultant to the U.S. Army's Bio-Sensor (Super Dog) program.

He developed techniques for training handlers for the U.S. government's General Services Administration and for guide dogs handled by people with multiple handicaps. He trained the first dog to assist a deaf person.

Captain Haggerty showed some of his dogs to their championships, and he is a former president of the Owner-Handlers Association, based in Long Island, New York.

He moved to California, where he now trains and handles dogs for Hollywood. He has more than 150 feature films and 450 commercials to his credit, and he writes and stages dog acts. He is a published author of more than 300 articles, and he wrote the dog training section of the *Encyclopedia Britannica*. He has won numerous awards from the Dog Writers' Association of America.

Captain Haggerty belongs to many professional groups and has served as president or as a board member for most of them. Among his credits are director of the Bull Terrier Club of America, Dog Writers' Association of America, Society of New York Dog Trainers, Professional Dog Trainers Association, Guild of Animal Theatrical Agents, Institute of Human Animal Relationships, Monterey County Dog Breeders Association, Bronx County Kennel Club and the Society of North American Dog Trainers.

Captain Haggarty lives in Los Angeles, California, where he has occasionally appeared in feature films himself.

HAMILBURG, DANIEL AND PHYLLIS. Breeders of Boxers under the Salgray prefix, the Hamilburgs were very influential in the breed for the twenty years between the 1950s and 1970s. They bought their first Boxer from Jane Forsyth, and in 1953 bred their first big winner, Ch. Salgray's Battle Chief. Through this dog and his progeny, well over 250 Boxers were produced, and the Salgray name continues to appear in pedigrees of the top dogs today.

HAMMARSTROM, SYLVIA. Skansen Kennels of Giant Schnauzers has produced more than 900 champions worldwide, a record in any breed. When the number reaches 1,000, Sylvia Hammarstrom plans to retire, but until then her kennel in Sebastopol, California, continues to flourish.

Hammarstrom was born in Stockholm, Sweden. She loved dogs all her life, and as soon as her parents permitted, she went to work in kennels and veterinary offices. Every summer her family went to their summer house to sail and to play tennis while she stayed behind to work with dogs. At a very young age she was allowed to work at some of the top kennels in Scandinavia, and by the time Hammarstrom was thirteen, she went to England to work at the Fred Curnows' Tavey Doberman and Borzoi Kennel. At fourteen she was in Switzerland in a Poodle and Papillon kennel outside Zurich and at fifteen returned to Tavey.

All through her teens Hammarstrom traveled the European show circuits, worked for groomers and veterinarians, building a foundation of knowledge that would enable her to start her own kennel with an excellent background in animal husbandry.

In 1960 Sylvia Hammarstrom emigrated to the United States, where she worked as an airline hostess. In 1962 at age twenty-three she was diagnosed with Krohn's disease, a debilitating intestinal disorder. Searching for relief she began her odyssey into nutrition, and she has developed a regimen that she claims has kept her healthy and active despite the physician's dire warnings thirty years ago. She continued to work as an airline hostess for the next twenty-five years while building up her kennel in Sonoma County, California, where she purchased land in 1964. She retired from TWA in 1986.

She resides with her large kennel of Giants on 100 acres, which the dogs share with a small herd of llamas and Hereford cattle. Hammarstrom has also bred Bouviers des Flandres, Rottweilers and Standard and Miniature Schnauzers. She is an AKC-approved judge of the three varieties of Schnauzers, Doberman Pinschers, Rottweilers, Mastiffs, Newfoundlands and Greyhounds.

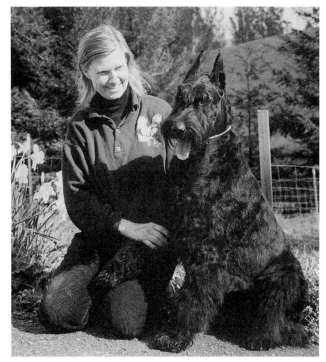

Sylvia Hammarstrom with one of her winning Giant Schnauzers, Ch. Skansen's Russian Roulette, photographed in 1996.

She has three passions in life: to show and breed her Schnauzers; to improve nutrition in dogs and people; and the theater. For the latter, she travels to New York and London to see all the latest shows.

HANSEN, DAWN VICK. Dawn Vick Hansen's involvement in the sport goes back almost sixty years when she made her debut at the first International Kennel Club show in Chicago, where she exhibited a Pekingese puppy.

In the late 1940s she traveled to England to bring back a show-quality Peke from a top kennel, but by a strange twist of fate a Brussels Griffon, not a Peke, made the trip home.

Serving in various offices of the American Brussels Griffon Association, including that of president, has been very rewarding for Hansen. However, her greatest rewards have been in her breeding program. Several Best in Show and Obedience titled Brussels Griffons have carried her Wil-Daw-Cy kennel name.

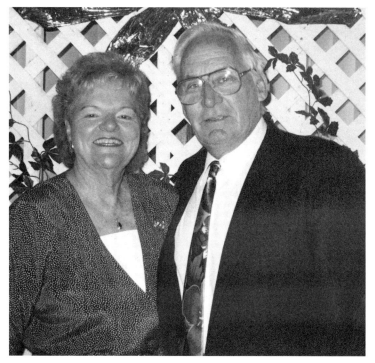

Dawn Vick Hansen and husband, Gil, breeders of Brussels Griffons. Mrs.
Hansen is approved to judge all Terrier, Toy and Non-Sporting breeds.

It was through her persistent efforts over three decades that the dis-
qualification against black smooths was finally removed from the Brussels
Griffon Standard. She was chair of the Breed Standard Committee and
serves on the Illustrated Breed Standard Committee and the Judges Education Committee of the ABGA.

Hansen and her husband, Gil, are retired and living in Wisconsin. She
has three stepdaughters and twelve grandchildren that make for a busy,
happy life. She admits to being an avid golfer but says her handicap is so
high she wouldn't reveal it.

When not practicing her swing, Dawn Vick Hansen can be found judging. She is approved for all Terrier, Toy and Non-Sporting breeds and half
the Working Group.

HARRA, FRANK W. Frank Harra became involved in the sport thirty-eight
years ago. Once a breeder of Collies, he was also a successful owner-
handler. He became an active member of the Collie Club of Long Island,

the Westbury Kennel Association and the Collie Club of America. He held key positions in these clubs, and he organized eye clinics and held conformation classes.

In 1970 Harra was approved to judge Collies, but his judging career was brief because in 1972 he joined the AKC as an executive field representative. Although he officially retired as a "field rep," giving up every weekend and several days during the week on the road, Harra continued to serve at the most important shows in the east. In 1996 he was appointed to the position of assistant to the AKC President Alfred Cheauré, with responsibilities to improve the AKC's link to the dog Fancy. His credentials for this position are well recognized and appreciated by the entire dog Fancy. In 1996 he was awarded the Langdon Skarda award, given to those in the Fancy who have made significant contributions over their lifetimes. In 1997 he was inducted into the Heinz Pet Products Hall of Fame.

Frank Harra served in the navy during World War II. He and his wife, Jean, reside in Blenheim, New York, with two Pointers and two Border Terriers.

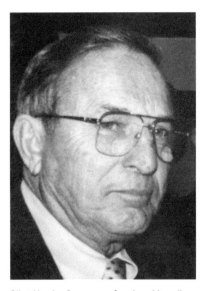

Clint Harris, former professional handler, now an all-breed judge.

HARRIS, CLINT. Clint Harris started his career in dogs showing in Obedience in the late 1940s. In the 1950s he established a boarding and training kennel in his home state of Kentucky and for twenty years conducted handling classes in Obedience and conformation.

In 1954 Harris became an all-breed professional handler, attending between seventy-five and eighty shows each year. He was one of an elite group of handlers who achieved Best in Show at Westminster for two consecutive years. In 1971 and 1972 he went to the top with the English Springer Spaniel, Ch. Chinoe's Adamant James, owned by the veterinarian Milton E. Prickett. During this time he served for five years on the board of directors of the Professional Handlers Association.

In 1980 he hung up his show lead and was approved to judge all Sporting breeds, and in 1994 he became an all-breed judge. He has judged in all fifty states, Canada, Bermuda and Sweden. His hobby is golf.

HARRIS, DR. DAVID O. Born and educated in England, Dr. Harris has bred and shown Bull Terriers under the affix Brummagem for twenty-seven years. He has judged Bull Terrier Specialties and championship shows in Australia and Asia, Great Britain, Europe, Canada and frequently in the United States. Harris judged the first Staffordshire Bull Terrier Club of America national Specialty and has also judged this breed abroad. He is currently approved to judge eleven terrier breeds.

An active member of the Bull Terrier Club of America, Harris served as president, and he chairs the Health Committee. He received the club's "Bar Sinister" trophy for outstanding service. He is vice-president of the Staffordshire Bull Terrier Club of America and its delegate to the American Kennel Club.

Harris contributes articles on the "bull terrier" breeds to books and magazines around the world. He has published a history of the colored Bull Terrier and has written another monograph on the breed.

Dr. Harris lives in Alameda, New Mexico.

HARRIS, LOUIS H. Lou Harris and his wife, Irene, have been active in the world of dogs for more than forty years. Their original breed was the German Shepherd, and later they bred both Pembroke Welsh Corgis and Afghan Hounds. He has been an AKC judge for more than thirty years and is approved to judge all Hounds, Working, Herding and half the Non-Sporting Group. He has judged at more than 1,000 shows in 47 states, Canada, Mexico, Australia, New Zealand, South Africa as well as in several South American and European countries.

Harris was president of the Blennerhasset Kennel Club in West Virginia for twenty-seven years and was an AKC delegate for twenty-four years. He has served as that club's show chairperson for many years.

He retired as vice-president of a major conglomerate in sales and motivation. He and his wife raise exotic birds at their home in Vienna, West Virginia.

HAUSMAN, DONA E. Dona Hausman comes from a longtime prominent family in the dog world. Her grandfather imported the first Saint Bernard into the United States from Switzerland. Her father's Airedale was Best of Breed at Westminster three years in a row.

Hausman's first dog was a Scottie, a present on her eleventh birthday. In 1937 she showed her Cocker Spaniel to its championship, and this dog became the foundation for her Meadow Ridge Kennel. She produced three champion Cockers from this line. In 1950 Hausman's husband, Jim, bought a Brittany, and she promptly finished his title as well. Two years later she did the same for another hunting companion, this time a Gordon Setter.

Hausman had always wanted a Collie, but decided to go with the smaller version, and it is with the Shetland Sheepdog that she has been most closely associated over the last forty years. She repeated her father's success at Westminster by going Best of Breed three years consecutively with her Ch. Pixie Dell Bright Vision. Vision also turned out to be a top sire and a great show dog for Hausman.

In 1942 Dona Hausman began to judge Obedience, and in 1949 she began to judge conformation. She is approved for all Sporting, Herding and Working breeds. She has been a guiding force in the Ox Ridge Kennel Club in the Stamford, Connecticut, area where she has been secretary-treasurer and show chair since 1955; for many years she served as its delegate to the AKC.

HEATH, CAPTAIN JEAN. The Black Watch Kennels of Jean Heath, a retired army officer, are renowned for top winning Miniature Schnauzers and Lakeland Terriers. Over the past twenty years Heath has been in partnership with the comedian Bill Cosby, and they have owned the all-time winning and producing Lakelands in the history of the breed. Her dogs have made great wins at the Montgomery County Kennel Club Terrier Classic several times, and Heath produced ten generations of outstanding Best in Show winners.

HECKMANN, WINIFRED. Winnie Heckmann was truly an all-rounder—breeder-exhibitor, professional handler and judge. She was born in Iowa, where her father raised Airedales and Dalmatians. At the age of ten Heckmann finished her first dog, an Airedale. She learned how to pluck and groom Terriers, and as a teenager she finished her first Standard Schnauzer.

As an adult, married with two children, she became a professional handler. After the death of her husband she moved to Maryland and built a boarding kennel, where she began to breed Irish Wolfhounds. During World War II she remarried, closed her kennel, gave up professional handling and turned to judging until her divorce in 1945. In order to support her children, she went back to handling and opened another kennel in Maryland.

Eventually Heckmann decided to give up boarding and handling altogether and applied for judging approval to judge all AKC breeds. She was considered to be one of the best arbiters of the day and was much in demand. Winifred Heckmann died in 1979.

HEITZMAN, GEORGE J. George Heitzman purchased his first boxer in 1951 and his first Doberman Pinscher in 1952. He decided that Dobes would be his breed, although he has owned a variety of other breeds since, including Siberian Huskies, Alaskan Malamutes, Afghan Hounds, Dachshunds, Whippets, Cairn Terriers, Boston Terriers, Dalmatians and Pembroke Welsh Corgis.

He served two years as president of the Western Pennsylvania Doberman Pinscher Club and began handling professionally in 1953. In 1985 he retired after thirty-two years. The following year he applied to judge and presently is approved for all Sporting, Working and Herding breeds, several Hound breeds and Chinese Shar-Pei. He currently lives in Fort Lauderdale, Florida.

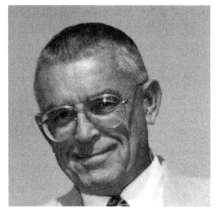

George Heitzman, former professional handler and breeder of Doberman Pinschers, now a judge of all Sporting, Working and Herding breeds.

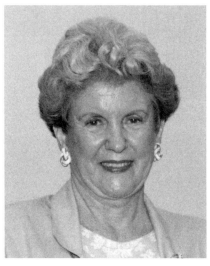

Barbara Heller once bred Weimaraners and German Shorthaired Pointers; she now judges all Sporting, Hound, Working and Terrier breeds.

HELLER, BARBARA F. Barbara Heller was born in Germany, where she owned Wirehaired Pointing Griffons, Irish Terriers and Pulik. After coming to the United States she bred dual-purpose German pointers and Weimaraners.

She has been judging for more than twenty-five years and is currently approved for the Sporting, Hound, Working and Terrier Groups plus eleven breeds in the Toy, Non-Sporting and Herding Groups. She has judged in all fifty states and in Puerto Rico, Mexico, Canada, South America, South Africa, Japan, Australia and New Zealand. In 1993 she judged Best in Show at Westminster.

HELMING, DAVID AND PEGGY. Pouch Cove Newfoundlands are recognized worldwide for their contributions to the breed.

Both Dave and Peggy Helming grew up with animals. Dave lived on a farm, where his father raised Black Angus cattle. Peggy was raised with Collies that were family pets. Both liked large dogs and originally set out to purchase a Saint Bernard. It happened that a famous Newfoundland kennel was across the road from the place they went to look. When they saw the big black dogs, it was love at first sight, and they came home with their first Newfoundland. That puppy was not structurally sound, and that experience led Peggy to pay particular attention to the health of her breeding stock. In 1970 they purchased a bitch based on Kitty Drury's Dryad breeding and several years later went back to the same source for another bitch. Those two bitches were the foundation stock for Pouch Cove, producing generations of top winning and top producing dogs.

Their first important dog was Ch. Pouch Cove Gref of Newton-Ark, ROM. A show winner himself, his greatest contribution was as a sire. His progeny, for several generations descending from him, have produced hundreds of champions that were the foundation of many kennels around the world. Gref died in 1984, but his influence is still felt through his descendants. Carrying on the tradition of great-producing dogs, multiple Best in Show and National Specialty winner, Ch. Pouch Cove's Favorite Son, ROM is today having great impact on the Newfoundland.

The Helmings' bitches have also been valuable in enhancing the breed. Starting with their first bitches, Ch. Kilyka's Jessica of Pouch Cove, CD, ROM and Ch. Kilyka's Becky Jo of Pouch Cove, ROM through to the present with Ch. Ad Lib of Pouch Cove, ROM, dam of eleven champions and Ch. Pouch Cove's Treasure Chest.

Both Dave and Peggy Helming have been active in the Newfoundland Club of America, serving on the board of directors and various committees and in their local Newfoundland Club, where Dave has served as president. They are also members of the Somerset Hills Kennel Club, where he was a show chairman. Peggy has worked with the Medical Genetics Department at the University of Pennsylvania on their studies into congenital heart problems in the Newfoundland.

Dave Helming is employed by an energy company in New Jersey. The Helmings live in Flemington, New Jersey, with about fifteen Newfs and a Portuguese Water Dog.

HERENDEEN, CHARLES. Chuck Herendeen was born in 1923 in Painesville, Ohio. He was raised on a farm and worked with all farm animals, including working dogs—hunting Airedales, Collies and Beagles. He entered the

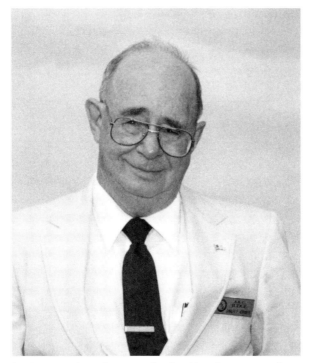

Charles Herendeen, former professional handler, now an all-breed judge.

U.S. Army in 1938 and spent more than eight years in the military with many tours of duty overseas.

Upon leaving the military he became a professional handler for twenty-three years, retiring to become a professional judge in 1973. He is approved to judge all breeds, one of the small number of judges to achieve that daunting goal.

He has been married to his wife, Rosemary, for fifty-one years, and they have three children and eleven grandchildren. They still live in Ohio.

HETHERINGTON, BOB AND JEAN. Bob Hetherington was enrolled as a member of the Bulldog Club of America by his father when he was four years old. He went to Yale, appropriately, and after graduation and his marriage to Jean, the couple bought their first Bulldog in 1962.

That was the beginning of the Hetherbull Kennel, which has produced about fifty champions, including the first UD Bulldog, handled by Bob, Ch. Hetherbull Arrogant Lazarus in 1975.

Bob Hetherington retired from the banking business, and the couple moved, first to North Carolina and then back to New York State, where they bought a kennel and enough land to keep their small menagerie of farm animals. Jean was the handler for the couple's dogs until she retired from showing to work for the American Kennel Club as a breed specialist. She divides her time between New York and the AKC's North Carolina office.

HODESSON, MARION MASON. Marion Hodesson was born in northern England, where her family owned a Collie and a Smooth Fox Terrier. When they moved to the United States, they brought a Collie with them, eventually settling in California, where they raised Collies with the Wilpshire prefix.

Hodesson began to train dogs, first for the blind and then for individual owners. She also assisted some animal trainers in Hollywood. She began to judge Obedience, and at the age of twenty-five received approvals to judge all Obedience classes.

She worked in a bank during the day and in the evenings at a veterinary clinic, where she met her husband, Samuel Hodesson. The couple owned and managed their own veterinary hospital.

Marion Hodesson turned to judging conformation and is approved for all Sporting, Working, Non-Sporting and Herding breeds. The couple retired to Tucson, Arizona, where they now reside. She is active in many organizations, including the Collie Club of America of which she has been a member for thirty years.

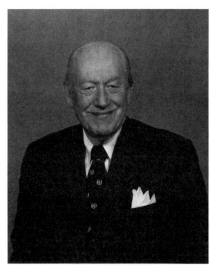

H. Anthony Hodges, Great Dane breeder, fly fisherman, woodworker and judge.

HODGES, H. ANTHONY. Tony Hodges became involved with purebred dogs in the early 1950s with a harlequin Great Dane that he acquired from the late Peter Knoop, while he was living in Canada where he was born. He later bred Standard Smooth Dachshunds.

He began his judging career in 1959 and moved to the United States in 1963. He judges all Hounds, Working, Terrier and Herding breeds. He is a member of the Westchester and Laurel Highlands (Pennsylvania) Kennel Clubs as well as the Great Dane Club of Western Pennsylvania. He is former first vice-president of the Great Dane Club of America.

Mr. Hodges is president of his own investment management company in Bolivar, Pennsylvania. He is an avid fly fisherman and woodworker. His other interests include vocal and instrumental music, photography and the cultivation of bonsai trees.

HOLLOWAY, D. ROY. One of seven children, Roy Holloway was born in Devon, England. At age ten his family moved to the United States and settled in Westchester County, New York. He loved dogs and as a young man went to work for the Pinefair Kennels in Greenwich, Connecticut. He learned to care for and groomed more than 140 Cocker Spaniels and Cairn Terriers in that position.

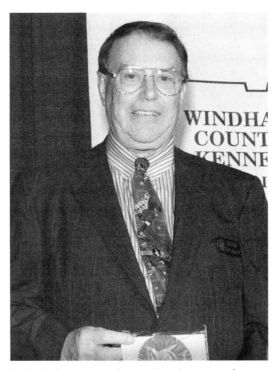

D. Roy Holloway, second-generation dog person, former professional handler and judge of Best in Show at Westminster 1996.

Holloway entered World War II as an army paratrooper with the famed 82nd Airborne Division. He was captured by the Germans five days after landing in France and spent the remainder of the war as a POW in Germany. After his release and return home he became an assistant to the renowned professional handler Tom Gately. In 1949 he and Bob Forsyth formed a partnership, where they traveled and showed dogs together for several years. After branching out on his own, Holloway built a very successful career as a professional handler until his retirement in 1982.

He became a professional judge and is approved for all Sporting, Hound, Terrier and Toy breeds. In 1996 he judged Best in Show at Westminster.

Roy Holloway has five children, one of whom is the successful professional handler, Doug Holloway, who won Best in Show at Westminster in 1997, carrying on the family tradition of great dog men. Holloway and his wife, Debbie, live in Reading, Pennsylvania.

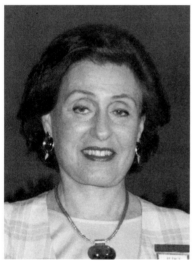

Evelyn Honig, student and collector of fine art, former Collie and Cairn Terrier breeder, judge and AKC delegate.

HONIG, EVELYN. Evelyn Honig was born in New York City and holds a bachelor's degree in fine arts. She is a docent at the Worcester Art Museum and is an avid student and collector of fine art in general and dog art in particular.

Mrs. Honig belongs to numerous specialty and all-breed clubs, including the Ladies Dog Club near Boston and the Worcester County Kennel Club, where she has held several offices. She has been a member of the Collie Club of America for forty years and is currently serving as the delegate to the AKC from the California Collie Clan.

With her husband, John, she has bred Collies and Cairn Terriers, and she is approved to judge the Herding Group and Best in Show.

HONIG, JOHN. John Honig was born in Vienna, Austria, and came to the United States at age fourteen. He holds a bachelor of science degree in engineering, and operates Angelo Fabrics Company, Inc., a fully integrated woolen and worsted mill in Webster, Massachusetts. He is associated with and on the board of directors of several companies, involving real estate and other investments.

With his wife, Evelyn, he has successfully bred Collies for approximately forty years and Cairn Terriers for twenty-five years under the kennel prefix of Accalia. He served two terms as president and twenty-three years as secretary for the Collie Club of America, Inc., and at present is director-at-large on his second, six-year term. Honig is a member of several specialty and all-breed clubs. He has served in all capacities for the Worcester County Kennel Club, where he has been the delegate to the AKC since 1972.

Honig is approved to judge all Working, Terrier, Toy, Non-Sporting and Herding breeds and Best in Show. He has been a judge for thirty years.

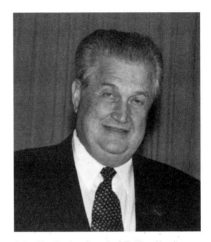

John Honig, husband of Evelyn Honig, former president of the Collie Club of America, judge and AKC delegate.

His hobbies, in addition to his involvement with purebred dogs, is a love for the ocean. The Honigs live in Worcester, Massachusetts, not far from the roar of the surf.

HOOD, DALE R. An Irish Setter and English Cocker Spaniel breeder since 1970, Dale Hood was born and raised in Baltimore, Maryland. Her main focus has been the Irish Setter, and she has bred and owned several generations of champions. She is a member of the Irish Setter Club of America, Potomac Irish Setter Club and Baltimore County Kennel Club. She is Secretary of Potomac and has been an officer and show chair for Baltimore County.

In her spare time Dale Hood enjoys collecting floral and wildlife prints, and she also is a master quilter, creating her own unique and beautifully executed designs.

HOPKINS, MARION. Marion Hopkins has been breeding and showing Irish Water Spaniels under the Mallyree prefix since the 1940s. She bred and owned Ch. Mallyree Mr. Muldoon, sire of the Best in Show winner and top dog in the history of the breed, Ch. Oak Tree's Irishtocrat. She also bred Ch. Mallyree Triple Expectation, CDX, JH, who was a Group winner as well as a Junior Hunter.

Hopkins lives in Bradford, New Hampshire, and is a delegate to the AKC from the Merrimac Valley Kennel Club.

HORN, DR. DANIEL AND JANET. Dan Horn was a psychologist, who was one of the first people to initiate studies that linked cigarette smoke to cancer. He was associated with the American Cancer Society, and in 1962 he joined the Department of Health, Education and Welfare, eventually becoming director of the National Clearinghouse for Smoking and Health. He spent a year in Geneva, Switzerland, with the World Health Organization and in 1975 moved to Atlanta, Georgia, with the Centers for Disease Control. He retired in 1978 to Frenchtown, New Jersey, where he lived with his wife of fifty-five years, Janet, until his death in 1995.

The Horn family's total involvement with the Chesapeake Bay Retriever started in 1946 when Dan brought home a puppy for Janet's birthday. They lived on the Maryland shore at the time, and their kennel, which has become synonymous with the breed, was called Eastern Waters. Since that time more than 115 champions have borne their kennel name.

The Horns' first big winner was a bitch, Ch. Eastern Waters's Tallapossa, CD, in 1961. Dan Horn's last dog was Am., Can. Ch. Eastern Waters' Break O' Day, Am. Can. CD, JH, WD who died in 1992. "Breakers" was the 1987 National Specialty winner, and he earned nineteen Group placements. Dan showed him in conformation, Janet took him to his Obedience titles and did all the field training. She handled him to his JH and Working Dog titles as well.

Janet Horn continues to show her dogs occasionally with the help of their four children and eight grandchildren. All the households have Eastern Waters's Chessies to carry on the legacy started by Dan Horn.

HOUPT, KATHERINE, DVM, PhD. Dr. Houpt is a veterinarian with a PhD in behavioral biology. She is a diplomate of the American College of Veterinary Behaviorists, editor-in-chief of *Dogwatch,* a publication issued by Cornell University College of Veterinary Medicine, and she is director of the Animal Behavior Clinic at Cornell.

HOWELL, ELSWORTH S. The founder and president of Howell Book House started his career in publishing as an assistant editor at the Grolier Society, publishers of *The Book of Knowledge* and other encyclopedias. He rose to become president and board chairman of Grolier Enterprises division. In 1961 he decided to combine his publishing experience with his lifelong devotion to purebred dogs, and he founded Howell Book House.

Howell had dogs all his life. His father, Clarence C. Howell, had a kennel of Schipperkes, and he bred, exhibited and judged that breed in the 1930s. The younger Howell had an English Setter as a boy, and it is

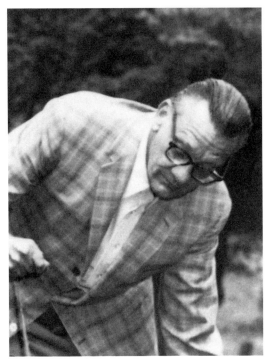

Elsworth Howell, founding president of Howell Book House, second-generation dog fancier, English Setter enthusiast and judge of all Sporting breeds.

with that breed that he was most closely associated. He bought his first show-quality dog in 1949 and exhibited many dogs with success during the ensuing twenty years. He also bred Basset Hounds, Dachshunds and Cocker Spaniels and owned several other breeds.

He was active in several dog clubs, serving as delegate to the AKC from the English Setter Club of America for many years, and he was a highly respected Sporting dog judge.

Elsworth Howell earned a reputation as a gentleman with wit and knowledge. He enjoyed his association with the dog Fancy and brought knowledge through the books he published to the general public in an educated, enjoyable way. He died in 1987.

HRITZO, Dr. J. ROBERT. A surgeon and chief of staff of a metropolitan hospital in Ohio, who operated a private surgical corporation for thirty-three years, Bob Hritzo is best known to the dog Fancy as the breeder of nationally ranked Samoyeds and Papillons and fifteen Bests in Show. The family's North Starr Kennels produced seventy-seven champions and fifteen Bests in Show. With his wife, Pat, and his three daughters, one of whom became a professional handler, Hritzo has been involved in the sport for thirty-five years.

He has been involved in dog clubs for many years and is delegate to the AKC from the Mahoning-Shenango Kennel Club. He was elected to a fourth term on the AKC board of directors in 1997. He is the corporate treasurer and was also instrumental in the formation of the Canine Health Foundation, of which he is the president.

HUNDT, TERRY LAZZARO. Terry Hundt became interested in dogs in 1963 when she purchased her first Doberman Pinscher. She had just graduated from Boston University and was teaching physical education in Massachusetts. The breeder of her dog was a client of J. Monroe Stebbins Jr. who was a top breeder and handler of Dobes. "Steb" thought her dog could

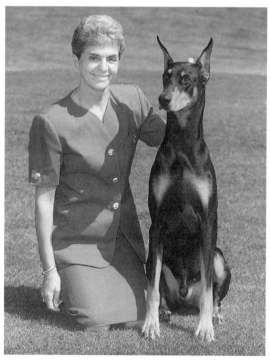

Terry Lazzaro Hundt with a favorite Doberman,
Ch. Ravenswood Rain Man v. Aquarius.

finish his championship and that was the beginning of a hobby that became a career.

During the years 1968–74, Hundt was teaching and going to shows and assisting Mr. Stebbins. When he retired to work for the American Kennel Club, she began handling on her own. She quit her teaching job in 1978 and became a full-time, circuit-bound professional dog handler. In those days handlers were licensed by the AKC, and she was able to handle Working, Hounds and Non-Sporting dogs.

She has had a career with many distinguished wins. In 1981 she received the Gaines FIDO award for Handler of the Year. She was also nominated twice for *Kennel Review*'s Best Female Handler award.

Hundt's career as a physical education teacher came about because she is an avid sports fan. She enjoys most sports, some as a spectator, some as a participant. Basketball is her all-time favorite. She has also taken up golf and hopes to pursue that hobby in her spare time.

HUNGERLAND, DR. JACKLYN E.

A licensed clinical psychologist, Jackie Hungerland is a native Californian, born in San Francisco. She is a graduate of the University of California at Santa Cruz and received her PhD at United States International University in 1980. She has a private practice in Monterey, where she lives, and is an adjunct professor at Golden Gate University in San Francisco. She is a consultant to the Visiting Nurse Association and has served on many professional boards as well as on her dog-related organizations. She is the mother of two children, Thomas de Russy Boyd and Margaret Boyd Andrews.

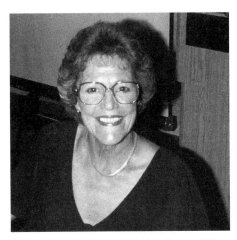

Jacklyn Hungerland, psychologist, former AKC board member, president of the Poodle Club of America.

She has bred Poodles under the de Russy prefix for many years. One of her most famous dogs was the great Standard Poodle, Ch. De Russy Lollypop, top dog of all breeds in 1969 and for seven years top winning Non-Sporting dog. Jackie has also owned and bred several other breeds of dogs, among them English Springer Spaniels, Dachshunds, Pembroke Welsh Corgis, Dalmatians, Whippets, Salukis, Maltese, Shih Tzu and Norfolk Terriers.

She is a member of Del Monte Kennel Club, Oakland Training Club, Poodle Club of Central California, Golden Gate Shih Tzu Club and Poodle Club of America. She served on the AKC's board of directors from 1985 to 1993, the first woman delegate to be elected to that body. She is president of the Poodle Club of America.

Dr. Hungerland has been judging for thirty-seven years and is approved for all Obedience classes, Non-Sporting, Toy and Hound Groups. She judged Best in Show at Westminster in 1995.

Dr. Hungerland has been a keynote speaker and participant at regional and national symposia and educated events. She is also a frequent writer in both her profession and in the dog world.

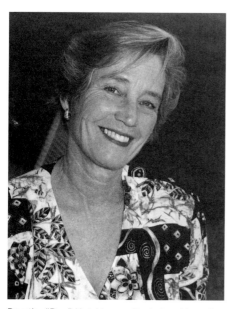

Dorothy "Dee" Hutchinson, Dachshund breeder, judge of all Hound breeds and avid sailor.

HUTCHINSON, DOROTHY O. Dee Hutchinson has been involved in the dog world for nearly fifty years as the daughter of famous Dachshund breeder Nancy Onthank. Her mother's kennel name, Rose Farm, is being carried on by Hutchinson to breed and show Dachshunds. She has bred more than 100 Dachshund champions in all coats and the two sizes, plus Golden Retrievers and Schipperkes. She has also owned an English Springer Spaniel, Bloodhound, Australian Cattle Dog and an Australian Shepherd.

She is a lifetime member of the Dachshund Club of America and was its delegate to the AKC until she retired from that position in 1991. She was a board member for eighteen years. She is a member of the Greenwich Kennel Club and was show chairwoman from the mid-1970s to 1993.

Hutchinson has been approved to judge since 1973 and currently judges all Sporting, Hound, Non-Sporting, Working and Herding breeds and half the breeds in the Toy Group. Her assignments have taken her to Bermuda and to several countries in South America and to Canada, Denmark, Australia, New Zealand as well as to most American states. She judged Westminster six times with her most memorable being the Hound Group assignment in 1995.

Hutchinson has been married to her husband, Bruce, since 1958, and they have two daughters and six grandchildren. When not in the center of the ring, Dee can be found sailing in the summer and skiing in the winter. The Hutchinsons live in Pound Ridge, New York.

She, with Bruce, authored *The Complete Dachshund* (New York: Howell Book House, 1997).

HUTCHINSON, LYDIA COLEMAN. Shortly before Lydia Hutchinson's birth her parents, Taylor and Esther Coleman, were given their first Cairn Terrier, and they exhibited a grandson of that bitch in 1949 to their first championship. Wolfpit Cairns was a family venture, producing 129 champions, top producers and multiple–Best in Show winners.

Although she is considered to be a senior judge, she continues to breed and show her Cairns from the home she shares with Dwight, her husband of thirty-seven years. In 1995 and 1996 she was recognized as the top breeder of Cairn championships as well as being the owner and breeder of the breed's top sire.

Lydia Hutchinson began judging in 1964 while still in her twenties, and she is approved to judge the Terrier and Toy Groups, Poodles, Giant and Standard Schnauzers and Cardigan and Pembroke Welsh Corgis. She has judged in Australia, Canada, Costa Rica and England.

She is a member of several dog clubs, including the Cairn Terrier Club of America, the Potomac Cairn Terrier Club, of which she is a founder, and the Columbia Terrier Club of Maryland.

The Hutchinsons live in Maryland, and their interests include antiquing, historic preservation and serving as docents for the local historical society.

HUTZMANN, ERWIN. Erwin Hutzmann was active in Irish Water Spaniels from the late 1950s through the 1970s under the kennel name of Naptandy. He came across the breed by accident at a time when few people were competing in the breed. His first dog, Ch. Shillalah Napper Tandy, CD turned out to be a Group and National Specialty winner and an important producer.

Hutzmann's line is behind many of the breed's most famous representatives, including Ch. Oak Tree's Irishtocrat.

He imported dogs from England and Ireland that, when incorporated into his lines, served to influence others over the years.

Erwin Hutzmann hunted with his dogs on both upland game and waterfowl and proved that the Irish Water Spaniel is capable of retrieving as well as flushing birds.

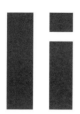

IRICK, MACKEY J., JR. Mackey Irick has been involved with show dogs all his life. He started breeding, showing and writing for dog magazines while in high school. Hundreds of champions descend from his High Heritage (Toy Poodles) and Rebel Ridge (Cocker Spaniels) bloodlines.

He is well known as the founder, publisher and editor of the *Poodle Review,* a magazine catering to the Poodle Fancy. He managed the magazine for thirty years from 1955 to 1985. He pioneered special stud dog issues and originated profiles of important Poodles. He was an early promoter for top producer statistics for dogs and bitches.

Irick is the author of *The New Poodle* (New York: Howell Book House, 1986) and was committee chairman of the *Illustrated Poodle Breed Standard,* which won an award from the Dog Writers' Association of America. He was also a member of the Poodle Club of America Publications Committee for *Poodles in America,* volumes 1 through 8. He is a collector of dog books, and his other interests include pedigree research and travel.

Irick is approved to judge Poodles and Cocker Spaniels, and he has judged at all-breed and Specialty shows throughout the United States.

He is a member of the Poodle Club of America, the American Spaniel Club and Dog Writers' Association of America.

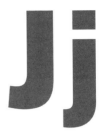

JACOBSEN, DIANE. Diane Jacobsen acquired her first Rhodesian Ridgeback in 1962 and bred her first litter in 1963 under the kennel name Baulenes. She changed the name to Calico Ridge in 1968.

Calico Ridge has produced more than 175 champions and more ROM sires and dams than any other kennel in the United States. Many kennels have used Calico Ridge dogs as their foundation stock.

JEFFORDS, KAY. A birthday present of a Boston Terrier from her husband, Walter, in 1966 started a hobby that mushroomed into a kennel of more than 100 dogs. Her Boston Terriers and Pekingese were important winners in the 1970s and 1980s.

The Jeffords are also deeply immersed in the world of thoroughbred horses, and their apartment in New York is filled with a collection of priceless artwork and bronzes of both horses and dogs. Walter Jefford's uncle owned the great racehorse, Man O' War.

Kay is a delegate to the AKC from the Des Moines Kennel Club, and she is an important supporter of the Dog Museum.

JENSEN, WAYNE AND MARLYS. Jen Araby started in the 1940s with stock purchased by the Jensens from top American and English breeders. They were particularly noted for their practice of importing good stock, taking into consideration both the pedigree and conformation of the individual dog. The Jensens were not averse to outcrossing and were successful in producing top winners in their period of active participation.

JOHNSON, DOUGLAS A. Douglas Johnson purchased his first Clumber Spaniel in 1984, which he showed and finished in 1985. His love for the breed and excitement for the competitive sport of dogs has driven him ever since.

He has shown three all-breed Best in Show winners and a National Specialty winner. He has bred two additional National Specialty winners and the three all-breed Best in Show winners. He is the breeder of Ch. Clussexx Country Sunrise, National Specialty winner and Best in Show at Westminster in 1996, the only Clumber Spaniel ever to win the top award at that show. "Brady's" sister, Ch. Clussexx Bubbleicious is also a National

Specialty winner. These littermates are the top winning dog and bitch in breed history.

Johnson has served as a member of the board of directors of the Clumber Spaniel Club of America, has served on the AKC Breed Standard Video Committee and was the CSCA's archivist for several years.

JOHNSON, R. ANN. Ann Johnson's Gold Rush Kennels was founded in the early 1970s, its bloodlines based on the top winning Golden of all time, Ch. Cummings Gold-Rush Charlie. Charlie was purchased as a family pet at the age of five weeks. He was not only a great show dog and ambassador for the breed but also an outstanding producer. His descendants are still winning and producing outstanding Goldens for Gold-Rush and for many other kennels throughout the United States.

JOHNSTON, SHIRLEY, DVM. A graduate of Washington State University College of Veterinary Medicine, Dr. Johnston made a specialty in theriogenology. For many years she was head of reproductive services at the University of Minnesota College of Veterinary Medicine. She has lectured to veterinarians all over the world about small animal reproduction. In 1997 she returned to her alma mater as the chair of Veterinary Clinical Sciences. Dr. Johnston plans to introduce the unique academic rotation for veterinary students that proved successful at the University of Minnesota with emphasis on the disease and genetic problems related to dog breeding.

JONES, JAQUE. Treyacres Kennels of Brussels Griffons is one of the most influential in America. Jaque Jones has been breeding and showing Grifs since the 1960s, and her most notable dog was Ch. Treyacres Zorro. This dog was the top sire in the history of the breed, having produced well over fifty champions. Zorro was also a Group and Best in Show winner.

Jones has served on the board of two Brussels Griffon clubs and was a member of the Breed Standard Committee for the American Brussels Griffon Association.

JORDAN, ANDREA. Andrea Jordan, with her late husband, Dennis, have bred and owned the top representatives of the Brittanys. Their Am. Can. Ch. Jordean All Kiddin' Aside is the top winning Brittany of all time with fifty Bests in Show and numerous Group and Specialty wins. He is the top producing sire in the breed with more than seventy-seven champions and several Field-titled offspring. Jordean dogs have dominated the top five rankings in the breed for the past five years up to 1997.

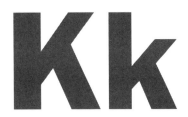

KAHN, GILBERT STANLEY. Originally from New York where he was active in his family's publishing business, Gil Kahn now divides his time between Miami, New York City and Newport, Rhode Island. With the support of his mother, Janet Annenberg Hooker, and the Janet A. Hooker Charitable Trust, Kahn devotes much of his time to his communities' cultural lives. He has had a long relationship with the Florida Grand Opera, serving on its board and executive committee for many years. He is also a former member of the Concert Association of South Florida's Executive Committee, was a former president of The Vizcayans and was very active with Fairchild Tropical Gardens. In addition, he is a major contributor to the Florida Philharmonic and a member of the Metropolitan Opera's Golden Horseshoe.

Kahn spends his summers at his Newport, Rhode Island, estate, Fairholme. There he is presently a trustee of the Preservation Society of Newport County, the Newport Art Museum and the Redwood Library and Athenaeum. In Washington he serves with his aunt, the Honorable Leonore Annenberg, on the board of Friends of Art and Preservation in Embassies. Kahn is also a member of the board of the National Museum of Natural History, where he has been very instrumental in creating the Janet Annenberg Hooker Hall of Geology, Gems and Minerals, scheduled to open in late 1997.

Gil Kahn purchased his first show dog in 1952, a Norwich Terrier. He owned Norwich until 1967 when he became associated with the Toy breeds. He bought his first Shih Tzu in 1968 and subsequently added Japanese Chin, Brussels Griffons and Chihuahuas to his Charing Cross Kennel.

He was the first delegate of the American Shih Tzu Club to the AKC and was also an officer and president of that club. He is presently delegate for the Japanese Chin Club of America. He has been a member of the Norfolk and Norwich Terrier Club since 1954.

Kahn is an avid collector of dog paintings from the nineteenth and early twentieth centuries and is the present board chairman of the American Kennel Club Museum of the Dog. He is also chairman of the Animal Welfare Society of South Florida and is one of the few American members of The Kennel Club in England. He has also endowed the Gilbert S. Kahn Deanship at the University of Pennsylvania School of Veterinary Medicine.

Kahn began judging in 1976 and has officiated throughout the United States and in several European countries. He has also judged in Great Britain, the Union of South Africa, Canada and Australia. In 1997 he judged the Toy Group at Westminster. He is approved to judge all Toy breeds, some of the Terriers and Non-Sporting breeds.

KAHN, KEKE BELBER. Keke Kahn has been in dogs almost all her life. Her breed was the Lhasa Apso, which she bred under the kennel name of Potala. She bred fifty-eight champions and six all-breed Best in Show Lhasas plus numerous Group winners.

She has been judging since 1972 and is currently approved for all Sporting, Hound, Working, Toy, Non-Sporting and Herding breeds and half the breeds in the Terrier Group.

She is married to Richard P. Kahn and has three children and seven grandchildren. Her hobbies are tennis, gardening, reading and dog club activities. She is particularly interested in judges' education. The Kahns live in Sarasota, Florida.

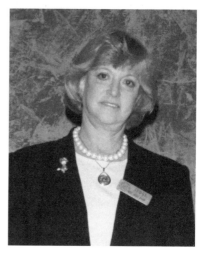

Keke Kahn, prominent Lhasa Apso breeder and judge of five Groups.

KANZLER, KATHLEEN. Kathleen Kanzler was born in Detroit, where her love for animals developed early. She has worked for veterinarians, at the National Zoo in Washington, D.C., and the zoo in San Diego, California. Her husband, Norbert, was an army officer and the family moved often. In the 1950s Norbert was stationed in Alaska, and it was there that Kathleen first became enamored of Siberian Huskies. She bought her foundation stock from Alaskan racing breeders, and over the years she has incorporated many of the top racing bloodlines into her Innisfree Kennels.

Kanzler bought her first dog, a Collie, in 1947 and decided on the Irish name, Innisfree, at that time as a reflection of her heritage.

In 1960 the Kanzlers returned to Michigan from Alaska and began breeding Siberians in earnest. Despite their travels overseas with the army, Kathleen was able to maintain control of her breeding stock by farming out dogs to loyal friends. In 1969 the family returned and established their home and kennels in Maryland. Because of their mobility, Kathleen Kanzler was forced to make hard choices about which dogs to keep as part of her breeding program.

Many dogs important to the breed were produced by Innisfree in the 1970s, but the most outstanding was Am., Can. Ch. Innisfree's Sierra Cinnar. Cinnar won thirty Bests in Show, considered a huge number at that time, culminating in Best in Show at Westminster in 1980. Cinnar was shown by Kathleen's daughter, Trish, who was the youngest handler ever to win at the garden, a record that stands to this day. Cinnar sired 118 American champions and many Canadian champions out of fewer than 60 bitches.

Cinnar's descendants have continued to produce top winning and top producing dogs for Innisfree. At the same time Kanzler has been true to her belief in maintaining the working qualities of the Siberian. She occasionally outcrosses to true Working Dogs, and she runs her dogs in local races in the Adirondacks, where she and her husband retired. Her daughters, Trish and Sheila, show the dogs, and Trish also works them pulling sleds.

In 1987 Kathleen Kanzler became interested in the Shiba Inu. She and her daughters have been to Japan eight times and have imported several dogs to use as foundation stock. To date, more than fourteen Innisfree Shibas have finished their championships.

Kathleen Kanzler has been approved since 1971 and judges all Herding breeds, Akitas, Alaskan Malamutes, Samoyeds and Siberian Huskies. She has judged in the United States and in several other countries. She also gives seminars on breeding, structure, gait, puppy selection and general kennel management. She has written extensively for dog publications and is consulted as an expert on the Siberian Husky. She appears in *Marquis' Who's Who in the World* (1996) for her accomplishments in dogs.

The Kanzlers live in Chateaugay, New York, near the Canadian border, a perfect climate for Siberians and Shibas.

KATSUMOTO, KAIJI. Kaiji Katsumoto was the first man in the United States to import a Shiba whose descendants were registered with a recognized registry in this country. This was done in 1973 with a dog named Nidai Akashiishi of Sagami Ikeda Kensha. Known by his friends as "Papa Shiba," Katsumoto continued to import quality Shibas from Japan for himself and for others. Today these dogs feature heavily in the pedigrees of some of the top producing Shibas in the United States. Kaiji Katsumoto and his wife, Toshiko, are still active in the breed, being founding members and the major force behind Beikoku Shibainu Aikokai, an American Shiba club with close ties to Japan.

KAUFFMAN, EDMUND J. In 1954 Edmund Jamison Kauffman and his wife, Sue, established Holly Hill Afghan Hound Kennels near Hubbard, Ohio. Their first champion came in 1958. Since then they bred and finished fifty-five champions.

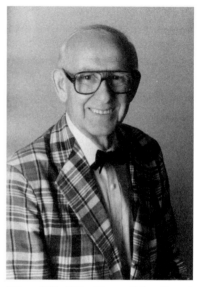

Edmund "Ned" Kauffman, Afghan Hound breeder and judge.

Kauffman graduated from Phillips Exeter Academy cum laude in 1934 and from Princeton University in 1938 with the same honors. In 1942 he joined the United States Air Corps and married Sue in 1944. He was assigned to the Eighth Air Force Battalion, 100th Bomb Group, and flew twenty-one combat missions before being shot down on July 28, 1944, over Germany. He was taken prisoner and liberated by General Patton's Third Army in 1945.

Kauffman was principal owner of a graphic arts company in Youngstown, Ohio, from the late 1940s until 1972, when he and Sue moved to Sarasota, Florida. The Kauffmans have three daughters, Paula and twins Sally and Susan.

Kauffman began his judging career in 1961, and he now judges all Sporting, Hound, Working and Non-Sporting breeds and Toy Poodles. He has judged at most major American shows and in Canada, Nassau, the Dominican Republic, Venezuela, Puerto Rico and Australia.

He is past president, show chairman and AKC delegate of Mahoning-Shenango Kennel Club, serving during the 1960s and 1970s. He is past president of the Greater Venice, Florida Dog Club, and former board member and honorary life member of the Afghan Hound Club of America. He has judged the Afghan Hound National Specialty three times and has chaired four educational seminars on the breed, beginning in the 1960s. He is considered to be an Afghan Hound Club of America mentor.

KAUFMANN, MRS. WALTER. Mrs. Kaufmann of Walhof Affenpinscher Kennels is credited with playing a major role in the perpetuation of the breed in the United States. All bloodlines of modern-day Affenpinschers can be traced back to Walhof Kennels. She also bred the first black-and-tan Group placing bitch and the first red male champion, thus preserving color other than black in the breed.

KAY, JANE G. As a child, Jane Kay's family owned Saint Bernards and Smooth Fox Terriers. As a teenager there were five Chow Chows and lots of Sealyham Terriers in the household. In the 1940s came more Sealys and, in the 1950s, Great Danes and Doberman Pinschers.

Kay became a professional handler and worked during the 1950s and 1960s, handling and breeding Miniature Pinschers, Beagles, Dachshunds and Doberman Pinschers, always owning a Chihuahua.

She began her judging career in 1970, which led to her being approved as an all-breed judge in the mid-1980s. She has judged in all fifty states and in more foreign countries than she cares to enumerate.

Jane Kay graduated from prep school in 1934 and from college in 1938 with a bachelor of science degree in education. She was married in 1941 to Harold Kay, who died in 1979. Their daughter, Carole, has two daughters, one of whom has presented Jane with her first great-grandson.

Her hobbies are golf, bridge and fishing. Jane lives in West Palm Beach, Florida, when she is not judging. She is a former delegate to the AKC from the Doberman Pinscher Club of America.

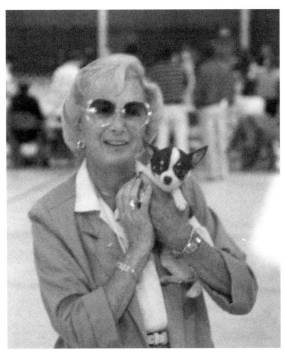

Jane Kay, all-breed judge, widely experienced breeder and former professional handler, always with a Chihuahua close by.

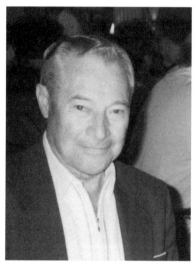

Nicholas "Nick" Kay, German Shepherd Dog breeder and exhibitor, Obedience and conformation judge.

KAY, NICHOLAS R. Nick Kay became interested in German Shepherds as a boy and had his first Shepherd in 1933. Since 1944 he has been attending dog shows as a spectator, steward, show chairman, "janitor" or judge.

Most of his professional career was devoted to work as a research chemist for a major oil company, but weekends and some evenings were spent helping others to exhibit, train and evaluate their dogs.

Kay was president of several Obedience clubs and of the German Shepherd Dog Club of Los Angeles County. He was also active in hosting the German Shepherd Dog Club of America National Specialty in the Los Angeles area.

Because of his study of dog movement he is asked to speak on the subject by clubs of various breeds. He started judging Obedience Trials in 1948 and conformation in 1951 and is now qualified to judge all Sporting, Hound, Working and Herding breeds. Judging in foreign countries is frequently combined with good snorkeling or hiking.

KELLER, G. GREGORY, DVM, MS. A graduate of the University of Missouri College of Veterinary Medicine, where he earned a master's degree in veterinary medicine and surgery, Dr. Keller is executive director of the Orthopedic Foundation for Animals. Dr. Keller was in private practice from 1973 until 1987, when he joined OFA as associate director. He is board certified by the American College of Veterinary Radiology and is an adjunct instructor in the College of Veterinary Medicine at the University of Missouri.

Dr. Keller has researched and written extensively in the fields of canine hip and elbow dysplasia and radiology.

KEMM, MARJORIE. A pioneer in bringing the Saluki to the United States and to encouraging breeders to breed and maintain their stock so it would be eligible for AKC registration, Marjorie Kemm imported dogs for her Anfa Kennels. A dog bred by her became the first American-bred to earn the international CACIB title. She was Ch. Anfa's Sarona and was a granddaughter of the late King Ibn Saud of Arabia's personal hunting hound.

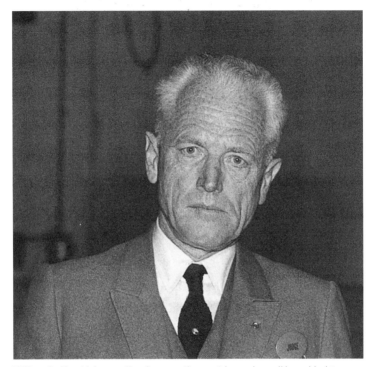

William L. Kendrick, one the dog sport's most legendary all-breed judges.

KENDRICK, WILLIAM L. Bill Kendrick, a legendary judge of all breeds, was born in 1904 in Ardmore, Pennsylvania. He attended Haverford School and graduated from Princeton University in 1926. While a twenty-year-old junior at Princeton, Kendrick began his judging career.

He was a Bull Terrier fancier, taking after his uncle W. Freeland Kendrick, once mayor of Philadelphia, and he later acquired the Queensbury kennel that his uncle had owned. In addition to breeding and showing Bull Terriers, Mr. Kendrick showed Manchester Terriers, Airedales and other Terrier breeds.

He was one of the few fanciers able to boast of having attended both the AKC's Sesquicentennial show in 1926 and its Centennial show in 1984. He was the Best in Show judge at the latter and an exhibitor at the former.

Mr. Kendrick was president of the Kennel Club of Philadelphia for thirty years when he retired in 1990, and he was also a member of Montgomery County Kennel Club.

He was a famous raconteur and enjoyed the company of dog people and judging. He died in 1992 and is survived by his wife, Vernelle, a stepdaughter and several grandchildren.

107

KNOCK, CAROL E. Carol Knock was a schoolteacher whose family hobby for more than thirty years has been purebred dogs. Her daughter, Lisa, participated in Junior Showmanship. The family has been training dogs in Obedience and conformation through their obedience school since 1965, and they have trained dogs in Tracking, Agility and Herding, as well.

Knock shows and breeds Belgian Malinois under the kennel name Tri Sorts. She has produced numerous champions and many nationally ranked dogs, including the top Malinois in the United States from 1988 to 1991. She was elected president of the American Belgain Malinois Club in 1995.

Knock's activities include match and sweepstakes assignments, serving as match chairman and being an active member of the Mid-Atlantic Stewards Association.

She loves cooking for family and friends, attending the theater, needlepoint, collecting antique prints and reading. The Knock family lives in Vienna, Virginia.

KRAUSE, ALVIN W., DVM, AND BETTIE. Both Al and Bettie Krause were born and raised in Colorado and lived there until 1991, when they decided to move to Henderson, Nevada.

Al graduated from Colorado State School of Veterinary Medicine in 1960. He started breeding and showing Miniature Schnauzers in 1962, finishing many champions. He handled the top Miniature Pinscher and the number two Toy dog in the United States in the early 1970s.

Bettie showed her first German Shepherd Dog in 1950. She was an all-breed handler and was fortunate in handling many Group and Best in Show dogs, including her own Best in Show Shepherd.

Both Al and Bettie Krause are AKC-approved judges of all Sporting, Hound and Working breeds. He also judges all Terriers and Non-Sporting breeds, Toy Poodles and Toy Manchesters. She judges all Herding breeds and Manchester Terriers.

They have judged in many countries around the world, including Australia, New Zealand, Japan, Canada, Mexico, Taiwan and several South American countries.

Since moving to Nevada they have taken up golf, and they both enjoy fishing and boating as well as just staying home.

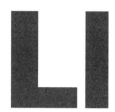

LAFORE, JOHN A., JR. Outgoing, progressive and friendly, Jack Lafore was the antithesis of Alfred Dick, the man who preceded him as president of the American Kennel Club. Lafore served as president from 1971 to 1978, when he retired. Whereas Al Dick was an autocratic man who never was afraid to raise his voice, Jack was the consummate politician, in the best sense of the word. Before he came to the AKC Jack Lafore served in the Pennsylvania legislature for four terms starting in 1950 and subsequently in Congress as a representative from Pennsylvania's thirteenth district from 1957 to 1961.

Lafore was a native and lifelong resident of Montgomery County in Pennsylvania and was an alumnus of Swarthmore College and the University of Pennsylvania. His working life touched on a wide variety of activities from the Bell System long lines operations in western New Jersey in the 1930s to founder and for twenty years president of an automobile dealership in Philadelphia.

During World War II he was a lieutenant commander in the navy and after the war entered politics. After he retired from Congress he became president of an aircraft corporation and then vice-president of a Philadelphia firm until he was tapped by the AKC, where he had served as delegate for eighteen years and on the board of directors for eight years.

Jack Lafore had been involved in dogs since childhood. His family had owned Great Danes, Saint Bernards and Old English Sheepdogs. With his wife, Margaret, he became a breeder of Collies, at one time owning 120 in their kennel in Haverford. In 1956 they acquired a Keeshond and gradually shifted their breeding program from Collies to Keeshonden. They kept as many as fifty during their most active years in the sport.

Jack Lafore is credited with bringing the AKC into the modern age. He was the first president to reach out to the Fancy with a series of symposia entitled, *A Day With AKC,* which brought the workings of the organization to its constituency for the first time.

Under his administration the most important change was the computerization of registration records. He approved a streamlined show award recording system, and he encouraged the revamping of the AKC publication, *AKC Gazette.*

Before Jack became president there were no directors of Field Trials or Obedience. He established separate departments for these activities, headed by people who had participated extensively in those areas of the sport before joining the AKC's executive staff. He created a position for a director of Visual Communications, which produced the first AKC films. This department eventually led to today's breed videos, which now cover almost every recognized breed.

The Executive Field Agent Program was launched by Lafore in 1973. This was the beginning of the involvement of the AKC into the investigation of unscrupulous breeders and its efforts to insist on compliance with the AKC's regulations.

Jack Lafore was a staunch supporter of financial aid to veterinary research.

He was an active member of many dog clubs in addition to the Devon Dog Show Association, including the Collie Club of America, Keeshond Club of America, Kennel Club of Philadelphia, Chester Valley Kennel Club and Westminster Kennel Club.

Jack Lafore died in January 1993.

LANDA, ELENA. Dogs have always been a part of Elena Landa's life. Her love of dogs started early. She grew up in a family that has bred and shown Bouviers des Flandres for thirty-five years. For the past twenty-five years they have owned a boarding kennel and grooming shop. Landa was always involved with the raising, training, grooming and showing of her parents' dogs.

Eventually she decided to have a breed of her own, and in the early 1980s she decided to concentrate on Soft Coated Wheaten Terriers. Her first dog became Am., Can. Ch. Legendary Baby Snooks, CD, CDX, TDX, Can. CD, TDX, ROM. "Puzzle" produced Landa's first National Specialty winner. Subsequently, her kennel name, Doubloon, has become well known for producing top Wheatens.

LANG, BILLY. Billy Lang was a drummer in a band for three decades and played all the big vaudeville circuits. He was a theater manager and a songwriter, and when he retired from show business in 1927, he became a professional dog handler, turning his hobby into his livelihood for almost twenty years. He was particularly successful with English Springer Spaniels and was an important mentor for Julia Gasow as she started her legendary Salilyn Kennels.

In 1946, Lang turned to judging, giving up his handler's license. He quickly became an all-rounder. In 1953 he became an AKC field

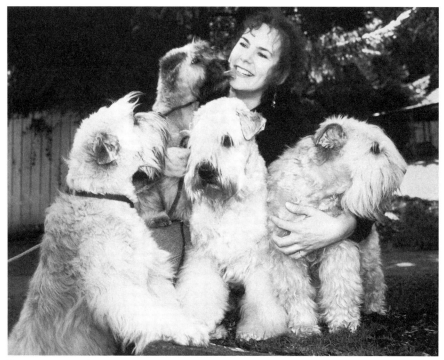

Elena Landa with four of her Soft Coated Wheaten Terriers.

representative. He was well liked and respected, with honors that include the Gaines FIDO award for Man of the Year.

LAURANS, PATRICIA W. Since 1963 Pat Laurans has shown dogs starting with Doberman Pinschers, one of which was a Best in Show and Specialty winner. In 1970 she began breeding and exhibiting German Wirehaired Pointers. Her foundation bitch, Ch. Hilltops S. S. Cheesecake, holds the record for top producing dam and is still one of the top winning German Wirehaired Pointers of all time. Under her kennel name, Laurwyn, many Best in Show, Specialty and Group winning dogs were produced and became the foundation for other kennels.

Laurans became an all-breed licensed handler and for several years worked as an assistant to J. Monroe Stebbins Jr. She attributes much of her devotion and concern for the sport and for the AKC to his teachings.

In 1969 Pat Laurans was involved in an automobile accident that was so severe that there was doubt she would ever walk again. It took more than eight years for her to regain mobility. The support and encouragement from people in the sport have been an inspiration to her and one of

111

the reasons that she became a founding member of the organization, Take The Lead, which offers assistance to those within the dog Fancy who are critically ill.

Laurans became an AKC-approved judge in 1981 and now judges all Working, Herding and Hound breeds as well as German Shorthaired Pointers, German Wirehaired Pointers and Standard and Toy Manchester Terriers.

Laurans is a 1961 graduate of Boston University with a bachelor of science degree in physical education. She received her master's degree in education guidance and counseling from the University of Bridgeport in 1969, and she has spent her working career in the Connecticut school system. She retired from her profession in 1995.

Active in several breed and all-breed clubs, she has served as the delegate to the AKC from the German Wirehaired Pointer Club of America for fifteen years. She was elected to AKC's board of directors in March 1996.

Pat Laurans is also a founder of the American Dog Show Judges Association and has been instrumental in organizing educational symposia in Boston, Chicago and Detroit for that organization.

In 1997 Laurans was nominated as Woman of the Year in the Heinz Pet Foods annual awards competition.

LAWSON, DEBORAH. Debbie Lawson has two loves that occasionally conflict in time and space. Most often she manages to balance both her love and profession of writing about and judging dogs and writing about attendance at performances of classical dance.

She was born and raised in Long Island and at the age of four announced to her mother that she would be a writer. While still in college she was offered a job at the Long Island newspaper, *Newsday,* where she filled a number of editorial staff posts, ending up as a daily op-ed page columnist.

She was married to the late Bernard Heyward Lawson, and the couple raised five daughters and two sons at the same time as they harbored as many as fifty dogs at their home in Old Westbury, Long Island. During this period Debbie Lawson freelanced as a writer, and after the couple moved to the suburbs of Philadelphia she joined the staff of the *Philadelphia Inquirer* from which she retired in 1989. She still writes columns and reports for the paper as well as for other publications. Her articles appear monthly in the major Dane publications in Paris, Tokyo, Finland, West Germany and Australia and occasionally in other countries. She is writing a history of the Kirov Ballet of Leningrad.

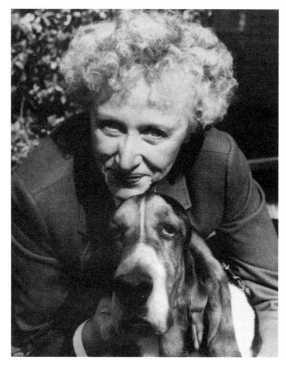

Deborah Lawson, widely read columnist and syndicated
writer, former breeder of Basset Hounds and Saint
Bernards and a judge of all Hounds and Saints.

Lawson was a breeder and exhibitor of Basset Hounds, Saint Bernards, Afghan Hounds and Bloodhounds for almost thirty-five years and is an AKC-approved judge of all Hound breeds and Saint Bernards.

She and her husband traveled widely, and she has been to the former Soviet Union (now Russia) many times in her pursuit of the dance. Her hobbies include needlepoint and decoupage. When she lived in Old Westbury, she raised and showed roses, and she used to enjoy fly fishing for Atlantic salmon in Canada.

Lawson currently lives in Strafford, Pennsylvania, a suburb of Philadelphia, where she pursues her active writing and judging career.

LEVY, DR. MARION J. Dr. Marion Levy, professor emeritus of Asian studies at Princeton University and his wife, Joy, are pioneers in the development of the Komondor in the United States. In the 1960s, unable to find one of the unusual dogs nearer home they contacted the Hungarian consulate and acquired a pup directly from Hungary. That dog became Ch. Szentivani Ingo, known as "Duna." In 1971 he became the first Komondor to win a Group in this country, but more important he was a highly effective ambassador for the breed.

The Levys were active in the Mid-Atlantic Komondor Club and the national club. He has been a delegate to the AKC from the Trenton Kennel Club for many years. He is a familiar sight at delegates' meetings and at the annual Trenton Kennel Club show, carrying one of his large collection of shepherds' staffs.

LINDSAY, NANCY. Lime Tree Kennels was founded by Nancy Lindsay in 1954 with the encouragement of her husband, Robert V. Lindsay. The Bloodhounds were raised at their home in Syosset, New York, where the Lindsays enjoyed a large collection of dog art and memorabilia. Robert Lindsay was a brother of the former mayor of New York, John Lindsay, and he was the president of the Westminster Kennel Club from 1969 to 1972. Nancy became a judge of the Hound breeds and before her retirement from judging officiated at Westminster as well as at many of the prestigious shows in the United States and abroad. The Lindsays eventually gave up their kennel and have retired to Millbrook, New York.

LINN, WILLIS. Edenglen Newfoundlands were among the breed's most influential families during the thirty years between the 1950s and 1980s. Starting with two Dryad bitches from Kitty Drury they bred more than sixty champions. Their bloodlines are found in most of the top kennels today both in the United States and several countries in Europe. They lived on the family estate in central New York's Finger Lakes district where Willis Linn had worked as an executive at Corning Glass.

LITTLETON, LEIGH. Leigh Littleton became involved with Borzois in 1974 and in lure coursing in 1975. When he and his wife, Judy, combined their Borzoi Kennels they combined their names coming up with Kalakirya Howff.

Littleton has been a lure coursing judge since 1980, and he currently judges at both AKC and American Sighthound Field Association (ASFA) Field Trials. He has been coursing chairman, treasurer and president of the Midwest Borzoi Club; coursing chairman and member of the board of governors of the Borzoi Club of America and chairman of the BCOA's annual national Specialty Field Trials in 1990, 1995 and 1997. He has been on the board of directors of the American Sighthound Field Association for fifteen of the last eighteen years. Of the many coursing hounds he has owned and campaigned, Zaraya of the Wild Hunt, JC, LCM XVII is the only dog of any breed to earn the ASFA titles seventeen times. "Locket" was number one coursing Borzoi in 1983, 1984, 1985 and then in 1988 as veteran. Leigh Littleton estimates he drove a minimum of 250,000 miles chauffeuring her to Field Trials, and he considered it a privilege.

When not engaged in the sport, he raises bamboo, bromeliads and euphorbia. He also develops computer software, which helps pay for the dog food, gasoline and fertilizer for his plants.

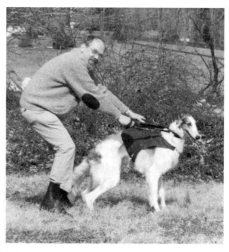

Leigh Littleton with one of his coursing Borzoi.

The Littletons live in Fincasts, Virginia.

LOEB, ERNEST. Ernie Loeb was born in Germany and knew many of the founders of the breed in that country. After he emigrated to the United States he became a breeder and importer as well as a professional handler of Working Dogs. He is one of the most respected members of the German Shepherd Dog Club of America and of the SV in Germany. He is a judge emeritus of several variety Groups.

LUCAS, WINAFRED. Srinagar, the Saluki kennel of Dr. Winafred and Miss Afton Lucas, was started during the 1960s with a combination of Jen Araby and English lines. The Lucases had a profound influence on the breed with their active breeding program.

Dr. Lucas was a clinical psychologist and was instrumental, with her daughter, in organizing the American Saluki Association in 1963. At one time Srinagar housed ninety-two hounds at the Lucas home in suburban Los Angeles and at a ranch at Lake Arrowhead in California. The population included Afghan Hounds, Scottish Deerhounds and Italian Greyhounds, as well as the Salukis for which the kennel was renowned.

LUST, GEORGE, PhD. Dr. Lust received his PhD in biochemistry from Cornell University in 1964. He joined the Baker Institute for Animal Health as professor of physiological chemistry and has been a pioneer in the study of hip dysplasia. He has published more than 100 scientific articles on the subject of hip dysplasia and osteoarthritis in dogs. In 1996 he organized the first scientific articles on the subject of hip dysplasia and osteoarthritis in dogs. In 1996 he organized the first scientific symposium on the subject at Baker Institute. His work is now focusing on the genetic aspects of hip dysplasia.

Dr. Lust has also published seven papers on the role in dogs of the pregnancy hormone relaxin.

LYON, MCDOWELL. McDowell Lyon's interest in dogs was a compelling force throughout his life. He was an outstanding dog authority and trainer, lecturer, author, judge of Field Trials, dog editor of *Outdoor Life* and for many years a staff member of *Popular Dogs* magazine.

It was while studying art in Chicago that Lyon decided to join the Canadian air force. Later he was transferred to the United States during World War I, after which he worked as an animal artist and copywriter in New Orleans. His work as a reporter led him to many assignments in the United States and abroad but he never lost his keen interest in dogs.

Among Lyon's most brilliant works in the field of dog writing that spanned many years were his articles on the study of conditioned reflexes at Johns Hopkins University. His analysis of the structure of the dog, the five senses of the dog and the gait of the dog led to his book, *The Dog in Action* (New Haven: Orange Judd Publishing Company, 1960). Ultimately acquired by Howell Book House, it became a best-seller in the field of basic dog books and an oft-quoted text on how dogs move.

McDowell Lyon died in 1959.

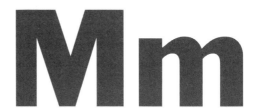

Mm

MACDONALD, DOROTHY. Dorothy Macdonald, or Dodie, as her friends call her, has been involved with dogs all her life. While growing up in England her parents had Welsh and Wire Fox Terriers plus two Golden Retrievers in the country. Her grandparents had Sealyham Terriers.

In the United States, Macdonald imported her mother's first Yorkshire Terrier for her in 1955 from the Stirkean Kennels. For the next twenty-five years she helped her mother raise and show Yorkies.

Macdonald has owned and raised Brittanys since the late 1950s, competing in both Field and conformation competition with an occasional foray into the Obedience ring. She has served as an officer and board member of the American Brittany Club as well as the California Brittany Club. She is now an honorary life member of both. Over the years she has written and lectured extensively on the Brittany.

In addition to the always present Brittanys, Macdonald has had a Champion Longhaired Dachshund and currently owns a Champion Nova Scotia Duck Tolling Retriever.

Dorothy has been an officer and show chairman for Malibu Kennel Club and Del Monte Kennel Club in California. Currently she is president of the Dog Judges Association of America and has been involved with its many symposia across the United States. She has been on the faculty of the American Kennel Club Judges' Institutes for several years.

She started judging Field Trials in the early 1970s and conformation shows in the mid-1970s. She is currently approved to judge all Sporting, Hound and Terrier breeds. She has judged all over the United States as well as in Canada, South America, Australia, New Zealand and the Orient. Her notable judging assignments include the Sporting Group at Westminster and numerous National Specialties.

An avid reader and collector of books, Macdonald has an enviable library covering several fields of interest, but predominantly that of dogs. She has more than 500 books dating back as early as 1781.

MACKAY-SMITH, MRS. WIN-GATE. Known by almost everyone as "Winkie," her name is synonymous with top winning, top producing Bull Terriers. She began breeding and showing her Banbury Bullies in 1968 and has been careful to give priority to health and temperament in her breeding

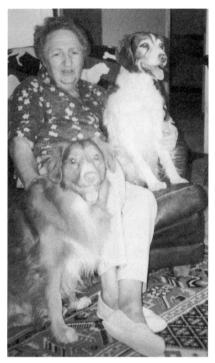

Dorothy Macdonald, breeder of Brittanys
and Yorkshire Terriers, judge, field trialer,
collector of rare books with her two dogs,
Ch. Millette's Lira Mac-Ben (Brittany) and
Can. Ch. Westerlea's Krugerand (Nova
Scotia Duck Tolling Retriever).

program. For the past twenty years she has been in partnership with Mary Remer of Bedrock Bull Terriers. One of her most famous dogs, Ch. Banbury Benson of Bedrock, was an excellent representative of the breed and a top winner in his day. His charismatic personality won many friends for the breed during his career.

In the mid-1970s Winkie became aware of a peculiar syndrome in some Bull Terrier puppies. Since her husband was a veterinarian and had been a colleague of Dr. Donald Patterson at the University of Pennsylvania School of Veterinary Medicine, she took some affected puppies to Dr. Patterson. With her help Dr. Patterson's Section on Medical Genetics attempted to identify and study the disease, called lethal acrodermatitis. The study was published in the *Journal of the American Veterinary Association* in 1986.

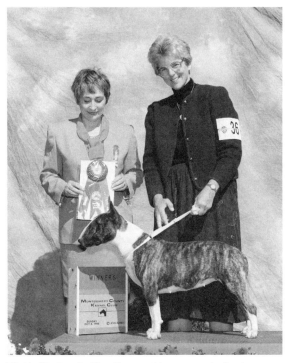

Winkie Mackay-Smith with one of her many winning home-
bred Bull Terriers.

Winkie's education was decidedly liberal arts. She attended Wellesley, Bryn Mawr, the University of Pennsylvania and the University of Delaware where she received a bachelor of arts in psychology and a master of arts in medieval history. Her hobbies include endurance riding, fox hunting and activities with her six grandchildren.

Winkie currently serves on the Health Committee of the Bull Terrier Club of America.

MAH, STUART. Stuart Mah, an oral surgeon by profession, has been involved in Obedience since 1986. He became very interested in Agility in 1989 and became a judge for several Agility organizations. He has given seminars for Agility exhibitors and future judges and has been selected twice to judge the World Competition in Agility. He represented the United States and AKC in Switzerland in 1996 on the first World Agility Championship team with his Border Collie. He runs a large Agility training school in Chino, California.

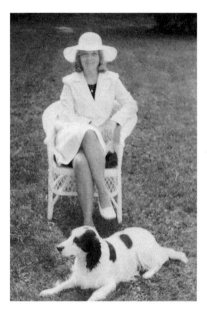

Jan Mahood, award-winning writer with her Springer-Border Collie mix, Kipper.

MAHOOD, JAN. Jan Mahood is a freelance writer and editor specializing in dog topics. Her articles on the sport of purebred dogs include profiles of leaders in the dog world, general information articles on conformation, Obedience and Agility, the human-dog bond, canine health and well-being, the dog in art and literature, training methods and legal issues.

She is the author of *Brutus and the Icon,* a general interest book about a homeless dog who becomes a hero. She edited *The AKC Complete Dog Book for Kids* (New York: Howell Book House, 1996), for which she wrote several chapters and breed sections.

Mahood also provides editorial and corporate communications services as a consultant to companies in the investment management and media industries.

She is a native of Long Island and lives with her husband, Gary D. Mahood, and two Miniature Pinschers on Shelter Island, New York. She is currently training one of the dogs in Obedience and Agility. Her other outdoor activities include sailing, swimming, kayaking, cross-country skiing and walking. Her favorite indoor activities are listening to classical music and jazz, curling up with dogs and a book by the fire or having friends in for her famous clam chowder or chili.

Her writing has been recognized by the Dog Writers' Association of America for Best Magazine article of 1995, and in 1996 she received the Alpine Denlinger Award for Excellence in Writing. Other awards have been a 1969 Virginia Press Association award for feature writing and a 1992 Financial Women's Association of New York commendation for organizing a series of professional development seminars.

Jan Mahood is a graduate of Syracuse University with a bachelor of arts in English. She completed her MBA with a concentration in finance at Adelphi University on Long Island. She has worked for various newspapers and magazines before turning to freelance work.

She is a member of the Dog Writers' Association of America, the Miniature Pinscher Club of America, the Empire Miniature Pinscher Club and the Dog Fanciers Club.

She has served on the board of directors of the Financial Women's Association of New York and the Prayer Book Society of the Episcopal Church, U.S.A.

MANDEVILLE, JOHN. John Mandeville has been an employee of the American Kennel Club since 1971. He is now vice-president of Operations in the North Carolina office. Before this assignment he was director of Systems Planning, assistant to the president, director of Public Communication, director of Judging Research and Development and vice-president of Planning and Development.

Mr. Mandeville attended the University of Vermont, San Francisco State University and Washington University in St. Louis to do doctoral studies on a Danforth Foundation fellowship. He is the author of the Dog Writers' of America's award-winning book *The Complete Old English Sheepdog* (Howell Book House: New York, 1976). He served on the board of directors of The Old English Sheepdog Club of America and was editor of that club's

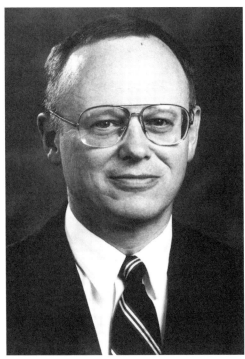

John Mandeville, vice-president of Operations in the AKC's North Carolina office.

newsletter. He and his wife, Mickey, were for many years breeders of Norwich and Norfolk Terriers. A litter of their breeding was the first Norfolk Terrier litter registered with the AKC, and a bitch of their breeding was the first to win a Group as well as being a Westminster Kennel Club Best of Breed winner.

The Mandevilles lived for more than twenty years in Montvale, New Jersey, where they were avid gardeners, before moving to Durham, North Carolina. They have one son, Henry, who was a top junior tennis player, an experience they say roughly equates to campaigning a special. John enjoys everything about food from watching cooking shows on TV to restaurants to cooking. He also reads everything from newspapers and magazines to pulp fiction, serious literature and non-fiction. He also loves movies on the big screen.

MARCEL, DONNA L. Donna Marcel has been on the editorial staff of *Dog World Magazine* for twelve years. She began at *Dog World* as assistant editor after graduating from Western Illinois University with a bachelor of arts in communication with an emphasis on journalism. She later moved up to the positions of associate editor and managing editor and was promoted to editor in March 1993. She has owned several dogs, including mixed breeds and purebreds. She lives in Bloomingdale, Illinois, and in her spare time enjoys in-line skating.

MARDEN, KENNETH A. A breeder, trainer and handler of German Shorthaired Pointers under the prefix of Crossing Creek Kennels since 1962, Ken Marden is a former president of the American Kennel Club, having served in that capacity from 1987 to 1990. He currently serves on the AKC's board of directors, class of 1998.

Marden has judged more than 100 pointing breed Field Trials and hunting tests, including six national championships. He has judged large sweepstakes entries at the German Shorthaired Pointer Club of America National Specialties.

He is a member of the Eastern German Shorthaired Pointer Club, the Diamond State German Shorthaired Pointer Club, Long Island German Shorthaired Pointer Club and the Princeton Dog Training Club.

Before joining the AKC he was employed by Johnson & Johnson, where he held a variety of marketing management positions. He then joined a Philadelphia advertising agency.

Ken Marden was instrumental in starting the Canine Good Citizen Program and the AKC Hunting Test Program. He continues to be active in both those areas and has also been a strong advocate for sensible dog legislation, testifying before local and state government bodies.

He and his wife, Judy, who shares his interest in both the field and show aspects of their dogs, live in Titusville, New Jersey.

MARSH, ARTHUR. Art Marsh, a retired AKC field representative, had a wealth of experience in dogs before joining the field staff in 1965. He was a delegate of the New England Training Club and a former president of North Shore Kennel Club. He was also treasurer of the Irish Water Spaniel Club of America. He became an Obedience and Tracking judge from 1953 until he gave up that aspect of the sport.

During World War II Marsh served with the U.S. Navy. He was born in Lynn, Massachusetts, and spent most of his life in New England until moving to Florida, where he was given the southeastern territory by the AKC. He became head of the field staff in 1978, and in 1991 the officers and members of the St. Petersburg Dog Fancier Club dedicated their show to Art Marsh in appreciation of his twenty-five years of service to the club.

MARTIN, DARYL. Daryl Martin has been in the sport of dogs all her life. Her parents raised and showed dogs, and she and her mother, Rena Martin, became one of the first mother-daughter handling teams.

She has handled many dogs to their championships and campaigned many different breeds to top dog status. Her charges have won the Quaker Oats award for Top Toy dogs on two occasions—the first in 1980 was the Maltese, Ch. Joanne-chen Mino Maya Dancer and then in 1986 the Shih Tzu, Ch. Cabrand's Agent Orange von Lou Wan took this coveted honor.

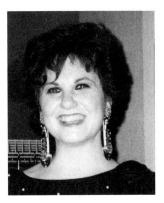

Daryl Martin, professional handler and breeder of Lhasa Apsos, Tibetan Terriers and Maltese.

Daryl Martin breeds Maltese, Lhasa Apsos and Tibetan Terriers and lives in Highland Park, Illinois.

MAULDIN, GUY A. AND THELMA. Guy and Thelma Mauldin founded their Shetland Sheepdog kennels thirty-five years ago, choosing Kismet for their kennel name. The meaning of the word is "fate" or " destiny." Many records have been set and broken by the Kismet Shelties, including breeding and owning more than 110 champions, owning 5 Register of Merit sires and 1 ROM dam. One sire and dam are the second top producing Shelties of all time. The Mauldins have owned many Specialty, Group and Best in Show winning dogs, with one of them breaking all records for number of Herding Groups and all-breed Bests in Shows won.

MAXWELL, ROBERT G. Bob Maxwell served as president of the American Kennel Club from 1991 until his retirement in March 1995. He was employed at the AKC for twenty-five years, starting as a controller in 1969. He was named vice-president of administration in 1985, senior vice-president in 1988 and executive vice-president in 1990.

He was responsible for the relocation of the registration and related services department to North Carolina, and he had begun the task of upgrading the computer system to handle registration matters more efficiently. He encouraged research into positive identification of dogs through DNA analysis and microchipping.

Bob Maxwell was known for his warmth and friendly attitude and his sense of humor. A longtime resident of Long Island, he now lives in Tuscon, Arizona, with his wife, Fay.

MCCAIG, DONALD. Born in Butte, Montana, in 1940, Don McCaig moved to Virginia and became a farmer and writer. He is the author of *Nop's Trials, Eminent Dogs Dangerous Men, Nop's Hope* and other books. He is a columnist for *Newsday, Dog World,* and can be heard on National Public Radio.

Since 1980 McCaig has bred, reared, worked, trained and trialed sheepdogs, particularly Border Collies. He is director and vice-president of the United States Border Collie Club. He led a spirited but unsuccessful fight to deter the AKC from imposing a conformation Standard on the Border Collie.

MCGINNIS, JEANNETTE. Jeannette can't remember a time in her life when she didn't have a dog. When she was very young she had a German Shepherd. Then came a rough Collie and a fifteen-inch Beagle.

She became involved in showing dogs in 1962 with an English Springer Spaniel, the first of many Springers in her life. She also owned Irish Setters, Longhaired and Wirehaired Dachshunds. Her first love, however, was the Springers.

She showed her own dogs for a short while but found out that a certain handler, Ray McGinnis, was hard to beat, so she hired him to show her dogs and she won a lot more! Ten years later he also won her heart and they were married. Together they handled professionally until their

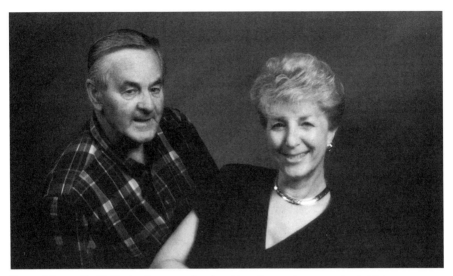

Ray and Jeannette McGinnis, former professional handlers and now popular judges.

retirement to judge in 1987. She is approved for all Sporting breeds and half the Hound Group.

MCGINNIS, RAYMOND, JR. Ray McGinnis was born in Washington, D.C., and at age four went to live on a farm near Warrenton, Virginia. During his school years he always had a dog, mostly Airedales, German Shepherds and Collies. For hunting he borrowed the neighbors' Basset Hounds and American Foxhounds.

He studied agriculture for four years and learned to judge dairy and beef cattle, swine, horses and poultry.

He served for three years in the U.S. Air Force during World War II. After the war he moved to California and became interested in obedience training. He owned Cocker Spaniels at that time and trained them for conformation and Obedience and enjoyed both aspects of the sport. He ran Obedience classes for twenty-three years and conformation classes for twenty years.

McGinnis became an all-breed handler in 1955 and showed dogs professionally for 33 years, making between 90 and 100 shows a year. First by himself and then in partnership with his wife, Jeannette, they carried between 15 and 20 dogs per show. He retired to judge in 1987.

Ray McGinnis is approved to judge all Sporting and Hound breeds and half the Herding Group.

Ray and Jeannette McGinnis live in Upland, California.

MCGIVERN, BERNARD E., JR., DDS. Bud McGivern started his career in dogs in 1954 when his mother, Jeanne McGivern, received an anniversary present of a black Miniature Poodle from his dad. The family lived near Cleveland, Ohio, at the time, and his mother immediately began training with the Cleveland All-Breed Training Club. Bud was about eighteen then and went along. His first dog show was the old Chagrin Valley Kennel Club show, now Western Reserve Kennel Club, at which he eventually judged twenty and thirty years later.

McGivern went to Notre Dame University and is one of the famous school's most loyal and staunch supporters. While there he began a little obedience training on his own and was ultimately put in charge of Notre Dame's two Irish Terrier mascots.

After graduation he attended dental school at Western Reserve University where he met a student nurse, Diane O'Neill; they were married in 1961. She shared his love of dogs, and they continued their involvement with Obedience, stewarding for trials in Ohio and Michigan.

Following his graduation from dental school, the couple moved to New York, where Bud began an internship and residency in dental surgery and Diane worked on her masters at New York University and began teaching at Bellevue Hospital. Diane has since received her PhD in nursing and has achieved a notable career in nursing administration.

While living in a small apartment in New York in 1962 the McGiverns decided to get a dog that they could hunt and show with not too much coat and small enough to fit into their accommodations. They decided on a Vizsla. Their first dog was a flyer, a bitch who finished in record time and became the foundation for their Bowcot Kennels.

Bud McGivern moved to Leonia, New Jersey, and then to Staten Island, where his practice of oral surgery was located. In 1965 a group of Vizsla enthusiasts formed the Vizsla Club of Northern New Jersey, of which McGivern was founding president. In 1968 the McGiverns helped found the Vizsla Club of Greater New York. Bud also has been active in the Staten Island Kennel Club, for which he is the delegate to the AKC.

McGivern is a member of the Westchester Kennel Club and Westminster Kennel Club. He has judged at both shows many times and judged the Sporting group at Westminster most recently in 1997.

McGivern is on the boards of Staten Island, Westchester and Westminster Kennel Clubs, Take the Lead and the ASPCA in New York. He also co-chairs the annual Handlers and Hackers Golf Tournament in Florida each January.

McGivern still shows Vizslas occasionally when he is not otherwise occupied. He judges all Sporting and Non-Sporting breeds, doing about thirty shows a year.

MCKINNEY, BETTY JO "B. J.". McKinney is the founder and publisher of Alpine Publications, a book publishing company in Loveland, Colorado, dedicated to the production and distribution of books that promote the knowledge and enjoyment of companion animals.

Started in 1975 as a self-publisher, the company now offers 150 titles on dogs, horses, cats and other animals.

McKinney has been a Shetland Sheepdog breeder since 1969 and is the coauthor of *Sheltie Talk* and *Beardie Basics*. She has bred, trained and handled Shelties in Obedience and conformation. She has served on the board of the Dog Writers' Association of America and the Centennial Shetland Sheepdog Club. She was newsletter editor for the Buckhorn Valley Kennel Club and is currently a member of the American Shetland Sheepdog Association, the American Management Society and the Rocky Mountain Publishers Association.

Before founding Alpine, Betty McKinney was senior publications specialist at Colorado State University. She previously worked in public relations and as a newspaper reporter. In addition to dogs and writing, her hobbies include hiking, horseback riding and reading.

MCKOWEN, ROBERT H. Bob McKowen of Leola, Pennsylvania, has served as vice-president for Performance Events for the American Kennel Club since 1988 until his retirement in April, 1997. During that time Herding, Lure Coursing, Agility and Earthdog events were added to the existing programs to allow more participation for those dogs and their owners.

In addition to the responsibility for those events McKowen's staff managed all licensed Field Trials and hunting tests plus Coonhound hunts and shows. To keep participants better informed, McKowen developed newsletters and seminars for the various events.

McKowen owned the all-time leading sire of German Shorthaired Pointer champions, and he served for five years as president of the German Shorthaired Pointer Club of America. He has participated in Field Trials and shows and has judged throughout the United States, Canada and Mexico.

Before joining the AKC McKowen was staff correspondent for United Press International and spent thirty-one years as senior press services officer for all commercial and industrial businesses for Armstrong World Industries. He is a graduate of the University of Pittsburgh.

Bob McKowen retired from the AKC in April 1997.

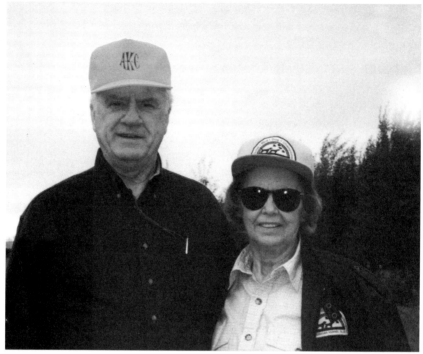

Robert McKowen and his wife, Lee. McKowen retired as AKC vice-president of Performance Events in April 1997. He is a breeder and field trialer of German Shorthaired Pointers.

MCLENNAN, BARDI. Dogs have been an integral part of Bardi McLennan's life. Her father had Smooth Fox Terriers in England and came to the United States with a kennel of French Bulldogs. In London during World War II, she rescued an American Cocker Spaniel from a bombed-out pet shop. In Edinburgh after the war there were Border Terriers. Back in the States in the 1950s it was Airedales, first, then Welsh Terriers.

Her Bardwyn Kennels produced several top winning Welsh Terriers during the 1970s and 1980s. Ch. Bardwyn Badger, now an elderly gentleman, was the last Welsh she showed, although she currently has a puppy from Wales, Felstead Fine Choice.

McLennan joined the Welsh Terrier Club of America in 1970. She held various offices, including president in 1984. Under her regime several innovations were started in the club. She is currently historian and newsletter editor. She was the founder of Glyndwr Welsh Terrier Club, a regional club, in 1976 and has been a member of the American Working Terrier Association since its inception in 1972. She works her dogs in Obedience, Agility and "go-to-ground," but not necessarily to titles.

128

Journalism has been her other life during all the years she bred and showed dogs. She was editor and columnist for Amy Vanderbilt for eighteen years. She wrote a daily column that was syndicated in 245 papers, plus a monthly page in Ladies Home Journal. She has written for many dog publications, hosted a local radio show about animals and produced a series of six audio tapes on dog behavior. She has written three books on dog care and a definitive book on Welsh Terriers, which is scheduled for publication.

MENAKER, RON. Ron Menaker is a managing director and head of Corporate Services of J. P. Morgan & Co, Inc. He is also a director of J. P. Morgan Services Inc., with offices in Wilmington and an operations center in Newark, Delaware.

During his professional career, Menaker has served on many boards of trustees or directorships. He currently serves as chairman of the New York

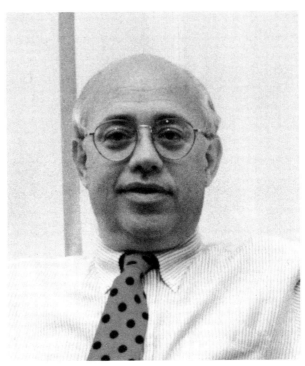

Ron Menaker, director of the American Kennel Club and of AKC's Museum of the Dog, judge and breeder of Giant Schnauzers, Bedlington and Norfolk Terriers.

129

Downtown Hospital and as a trustee of the New York University Medical Center. He is a director and past president of the AKC's Museum of the Dog and a trustee of St. Hubert's Giralda Animal Welfare and Education Center. He is a former trustee of the Morris Animal Foundation.

Ron Menaker was appointed director of the American Kennel Club in 1996 to fill an unexpired term and was re-elected to a one-year unexpired term in 1997. He is the delegate to the AKC from the Des Moines Obedience Training Club. For the past eight years he has been show chairman for the Westminster Kennel Club.

He is a member of several specialty and all-breed clubs, including the Bedlington Terrier Club of America, where he has held various positions, including president, director and delegate.

Menaker has been actively involved in the sport of purebred dogs for more than thirty years. He has bred and exhibited Giant Schnauzers, Bedlington Terriers and Norfolk Terriers. A licensed judge since 1994, he judges eleven Working breeds and two Terrier breeds. An avid collector of sporting art, Menaker resides in Wyckoff, New Jersey.

MERRIAM, HON. DAVID. Dave Merriam has been in the dog sport for forty-five years, breeding, exhibiting and judging Bull Terriers. He received his first dog as a gift when he was fourteen years old. At present he is the president of the Bull Terrier Club of America and chairman of the board of directors of the American Kennel Club. He serves as delegate from the Duluth Kennel Club.

Judge Merriam has had a long history of service to the AKC. He was first appointed to the board in 1979 and was twice elected to that position, resigning in 1986. He returned to the board in 1994, and later served as chief operating officer of the AKC in an interim capacity. In 1997 he was again elected to the board for a four-year term, becoming chairman.

A graduate of UCLA Law School with a master's from Stanford in political science, Judge Merriam started his career as a deputy district attorney and later worked in private practice for four years. He served as a municipal court judge for San Bernadino County, California, for twenty years, retiring from that position in 1993.

As an AKC board member, Merriam was instrumental in getting the delegate body more involved in kennel club deliberations through the establishment of delegate committees.

He has been approved to judge Terriers since 1966. When not officiating in the ring or occasionally exhibiting his Broadside Bull Terriers, Judge Merriam enjoys traveling to exotic places. He resides in Upland, California.

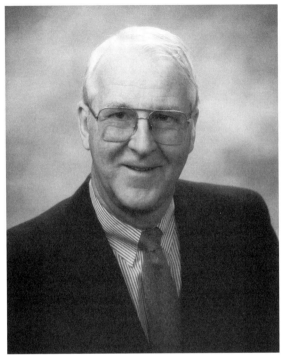

Hon. David Merriam, American Kennel Club's chairman of the board, judge of all Terriers.

MEYER, DICK AND CAROL A. Dick and Carol Meyer are the owners of Starhaven French Bulldogs. As owner-handlers they have been showing their dogs since 1987, producing Group, Specialty and Best in Show winners.

They are charter members of the Hoosier Rottweiler Club, and Carol is show chairwoman for the Central Indiana Kennel Club. The Meyers enjoy creativity with stained glass and crafts. Carol is a gourmet cook and does cake decorating and candy making. They live in Indianapolis, Indiana.

MILLER, FRED T. Fred Miller is president and chief executive officer of the United Kennel Club, Inc. He has been associated with dogs all his life. He has raised both Sealyham Terriers and Basset Hounds.

During his twenty-four year tenure with the UKC he has broadened the scope of this registry to develop friendly, education-based owner-handler programs. He has encouraged development of Coonhound championship events and Obedience and conformation events. His

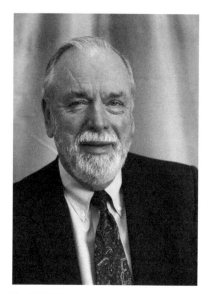

Fred T. Miller, president and CEO of the United Kennel Club.

organization was the first to use DNA technology for registration identification. His registry was the first to establish a "puppy mill program," designed to eliminate unscrupulous breeders from the registry.

He is a member of the American Dog Owners Association and is vice-president of its Canine Defense Fund. Mr. Miller is past director of the United Conservation Alliance, Inc., and in the last fifteen years has been extremely active in combating breed-specific legislation throughout the country.

Fred Miller has three children. His wife is the former Connie Gerstner, who was a professional handler and breeder of Golden Retrievers under the Malagold prefix. They reside in Kalamazoo, Michigan, where they raise and show Golden Retrievers. He is past president of the Kalamazoo Rotary Club, past president of the Park Club of Kalamazoo and a member of the First United Methodist Church. He is also a member of the Dog Writers' Association of America, where he sponsors the annual "Communicators Award."

MOHR, ALICIA. Kimani Rhodesian Ridgeback Kennels began in 1963 with Mohr's first home-bred champion, Weecha's Kimani of Mohrridge. Since then she has produced 175 champions, including 8 National Specialty Bests of Breed, many Best in Show winners and Obedience titlists.

Alicia Mohr is past president of the Rhodesian Ridgeback Club of the United States. She is also an international judge, most recently having been honored with the South African Rhodesian Ridgeback Club Specialty assignment. She lives with her husband, John, in Chester, New Jersey.

MOORE, BETTY COX. Betty Moore is a native of Sommerville, Texas, the mother of two children and grandmother of two. She and her husband, Norton, became active in dogs in 1957. They were breeders and exhibitors of Doberman Pinschers and Miniature Pinschers. She became an all-breed handler, a profession she followed until 1976, when she began to judge. She is currently approved for all Working, Terrier, Toy, Non-Sporting and

Herding breeds, as well as for some Sporting dogs and Hounds. In 1997 she judged the Herding Group at Westminster. Norton is approved to judge all Sporting and Hound breeds and some of the Working breeds. The couple live in Houston, Texas, where Betty is a founding member of the Doberman Pinscher Club of Houston.

MOORE, ROBERT J. Bob Moore started his purebred dog activities with Boxers about fifty years ago. His first champion was Mazelaine's Hot Shot, a son of the immortal Brandy. In 1951 he became involved in Miniature Schnauzers and bred several champions under the Bethel's prefix. He also owned and finished dogs of several other breeds.

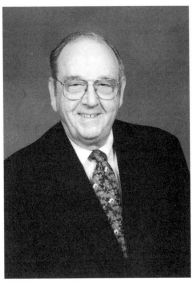

Moore is retired as a sales representative for Kraft, Inc. He and his wife, Gene, live in Decatur, Georgia. They have two sons and five grandchildren.

He began judging in 1961 and became an all-rounder in 1990. He has judged in all fifty states, Puerto Rico, Sweden, most of the Canadian provinces and in Australia three times.

Robert J. Moore, all-breed judge and former breeder of Boxers and Miniature Schnauzers.

His hobbies include playing the organ, genealogy, mall walking and, of course, dogs. He now has a thirteen-year-old Australian Cattle Dog, which is the top Register of Merit Sire in the United States, and a wonderful, half-eared, undershot, neutered Dandie Dinmont Terrier, known far and wide as Vinnie.

MORRIS, MARK L., JR., DVM, PhD. Dr. Morris received his DVM from Cornell University in 1958 and his PhD in veterinary pathology and nutrition from the University of Wisconsin in 1963. Dr. Morris is one of the nation's outstanding companion animal nutritionists.

He is carrying on work pioneered by his father in this field. His dietary foods are found throughout the world and have been used for more than forty-five years in maintaining pets with a variety of diseases. While he is best known as the developer of Science Diet™ pet foods, his specialized products have been fed to sled dogs in Antarctica and air-dropped to guard dogs in Southeast Asia.

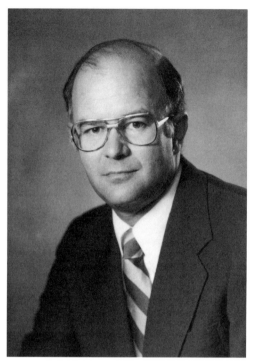

Mark L. Morris, Jr., DVM, PhD, research vice-president of Morris Animal Foundation and a veterinary nutritionist.

His revolutionary approach to zoo nutrition has rewritten the book on endangered species conservation.

Dr. Morris has served as editor of sections on nutrition in *Current Veterinary Therapy,* the *Cornell Book of Cats,* and *Canine Medicine.* He has contributed articles to numerous veterinary texts and is coauthor of the textbook, *Small Animal Clinical Nutrition 3.*

Dr. Morris is a charter diplomate of the American College of Veterinary Nutrition. He serves as research vice-president of the Morris Animal Foundation, a nonprofit foundation started by his father, which works to improve the health of dogs, cats, horses, zoo animals and wildlife by funding health studies and providing education to veterinarians, breeders and pet owners.

MOUAT, HUGH R., DVM. A veterinarian located in Amsterdam, New York, Dr. Mouat is credited with launching the real beginning of Otter Hound breeding in the United States. In 1940 he acquired his foundation stock and in 1956 began using the kennel name, Adriucha, an Indian word meaning "valiant one." Adriucha appears in all pedigrees of totally American-bred Otter Hounds. His early breeding program suffered many setbacks because of disease and blood disorders. With advances in veterinary medicine the number of puppy losses in his kennel declined, and Dr. Mouat sought the help of W. Jean Dodds, DVM, to unravel a bleeding disorder that affected his stock. Dr. Dodds found a platelet function defect, and in 1966 blood testing on his hounds was begun. Through careful selection, Dr. Mouat was able to eliminate the disease from his breeding stock.

In 1970 Dr. Mouat was honored by the Otter Hound Club of America for his thirty-five years of service. He died in 1981, but before his death he gave much of his extensive collection of Otter Hound books and art to the library at Cornell University School of Veterinary Medicine.

MOUNCE, DENNY. A native of Houston and a fourth generation Texan, Denny Mounce has been involved in dogs for forty years.

She is a graduate of Greenbrier College, majoring in liberal arts. She majored in animal science at Texas A & M and was a marketing student at North Harris College.

Her first purebred dog was a West Highland White Terrier in 1954. As a teen and a young adult she worked as a veterinary assistant while attending school.

Mounce began handling as an assistant in 1973 with Sporting dogs. She began her interest in Dachshunds in 1975 and with partner, Peggy Lloyd, bred and showed some of the top winning and producing Miniature Wirehaired Dachshunds in America. Of particular fame were Ch. Daiquiri's Fanny Farkle, MW, the top winning bitch in the history of the breed and Ch. Cal-Neva's Hy Tymes, MW, who produced twelve champions carrying Mounce's Pegden prefix.

In 1978 she received her license as a professional handler, and over the next twenty years she and Peggy won nearly 100 Bests in Show, Groups and Group placements showing dogs in all seven Groups.

In 1988 she received the first of five consecutive nominations for *Kennel Review*'s Best Female Professional Handler. In 1989, 1990 and 1992 she won that award, making her the first handler to be inducted into the *Kennel Review* Hall of Fame.

She was a Certified Professional Handler and an active member of the Dog Handlers Guild.

Denny continues to show dogs, though she has trimmed her work schedule. Most recently, Denny Mounce retired from the handling profession to pursue a judging career.

MURPHY, CATHERINE M. Kitty Murphy and her late husband, Fred, acquired their first Brittany in 1959. Since then she has done limited breeding, but her dogs have had a major impact on the breed. In the 1970s Ch. AFC Sequani's Dana MacDuff, bred and shown by Murphy, won forty-four Group placements and sired forty-six show champions. In those days, Brittanys almost never placed in the Sporting Groups. Duffy's son, Ch. Blazer Sequani Maximilian, owned by Kuno Spies, won several Groups and a Best in Show. The last of Duffy's offspring was Squire. He went to fewer than twenty shows in his lifetime and at the age of eleven was entered as a veteran in the Maryland Specialty. He defeated sixty-five Brittanys that day and went on to win the Group and Best in Show. Squire was broken to the field at nine years of age and went on to win five placements in the one season he was campaigned.

Murphy served as AKC delegate from the American Brittany Club for eight years and president for two terms. She was elected to the Brittany Club Hall of Fame. She was vice-president of the Michigan Brittany Club and during the time she lived in New Jersey served as president, vice-president and treasurer of the North Jersey Brittany Club, where she is a life member. She has been a member of Somerset Hills Kennel Club since 1967, serving as president and delegate and is now a life member.

Murphy retired to Yorktown, Virginia, several years ago, but never misses the Brittany Club National Specialty and Field Trial held in Arkansas in November.

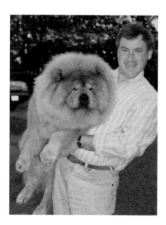

Desmond "Desi" Murphy with one of his top winning Chow Chows, Ch. Luv-Chow's Risen Star.

MURPHY, DESMOND J. Desi Murphy was born in Scotland on December 2, 1948. At the age of six months his family moved to Huntington, New York, where his father, Harry, a well-known dog man and handler managed an Airedale Kennel for Mr. and Mrs. William Buckley. Mr. Buckley was at that time president of the American Kennel Club.

From age two, Desi Murphy's life was spent living at the Mardormere Kennels in Old Brookville, New York, with large numbers of Whippets and Greyhounds. During that time he raised Norwich Terriers on his own. When he was six, he started going to dog shows with his father, and he has been attending dog events ever since.

In his early teens he spent more time working with his uncle John Murphy, a distinguished Terrier handler who became an all-round judge. Murphy worked for many different handlers on weekends, and while in high school and college he worked part-time for the AKC.

He continued to exhibit his own dogs and in 1967 formed a partnership with Dr. Sam Draper that has lasted thirty years. Their Liontamer Chows produced six Best in Show winners. In 1972 he started judging and is approved to judge fifty-two breeds in six Groups, including all Terriers.

Desi Murphy is a dental products salesman. His other interests involve searching for fine restaurants and spending "quality time" with dog friends.

MURR, LOUIS. A major figure in the dog world for fifty-six years, Louis Murr was famous as a breeder, exhibitor and judge. His Romanoff Kennels held as many as ninety Borzoi, with the best being Ch. Vigow of Romanoff.

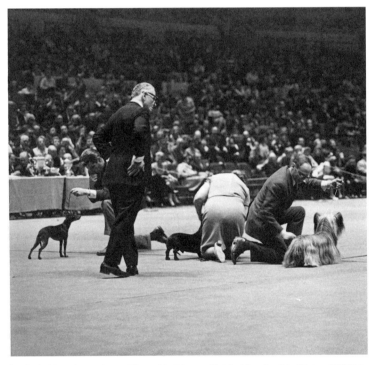

Louis J. Murr, legendary all-breed judge scrutinizing the Best in Show eligibles at the 1969 Westminster show. He ultimately selected the Skye Terrier Ch. Glamoor Good News, handled by her owner Walter F. Goodman, whose biography appears in an earlier chapter.

Mr. Murr was born in the Basque country, came to the United States as a youngster and served in the U.S. Army in World War I. He opened an antique shop in New York City and in 1920 attended his first dog show, Westminster.

Louis Murr and Westminster were a regular feature. His name appeared on the panel for twenty-one consecutive years, and in 1969 he judged Best in Show. His last show was in 1976 at age eighty-two in Vineland, New Jersey. He passed away shortly thereafter in February 1978.

MURRAY, ROY. Roy Murray's father and mother were professional handlers, and he carried on the tradition. His father, Lee, became an all-breed judge. Roy is a Certified Professional Handler and a member of the Dog Handlers Guild.

He has shown many top winning dogs, including two of the most prominent German Shorthaired Pointers in the breed. He also piloted a top Standard Smooth Dachshund and a two-time winner of the Quaker Oats award, a Samoyed, Ch. Quicksilver Razz Ma Tazz, who also twice won the National Specialty.

Roy Murray is a member of the Fort Worth Kennel Club and the Irish Setter Club of Fort Worth. He and his wife, Shirlee, live in Roanoke, Texas.

MURRAY, SHIRLEE. Shirlee Murray started in dogs in 1973, breeding Irish Setters under the Kennlee prefix. She became an all-breed professional handler and has piloted more than 100 Irish Setters of her own breeding and that of her clients to their championships and numerous Bests in Show. She has also shown the top Pharoah Hound in that breed's history and a record-breaking Brittany as well.

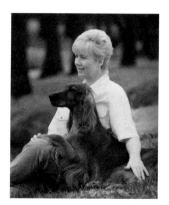

Shirlee Murray, breeder of Irish Setters and with her husband, Roy, professional handler.

Shirlee Murray is a board-certified professional handler and a member of the Dog Handlers' Guild. She and her husband, Roy, continue their careers as professional handlers from their kennel and home in Roanoke, Texas.

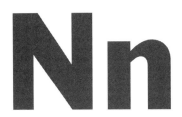

Nn

NEFF, JOHN C. John C. Neff was an Irish Setter breeder who was a delegate for the Irish Setter Club of America from 1942 to 1977. He became executive vice-president of the AKC in 1951 and served in that capacity until 1964. Under his administration a pension plan for employees was started, improvements to the Stud Book and registration procedures were begun, including microfilming of early records, and he instigated the move from the AKC's cramped quarters on Park Avenue South to Madison Avenue. He died in 1982.

NELSON, HOLLY J., DVM. Dr. Nelson is well known for her research concerning Dalmatians. She collaborated with scientists at the University of California at Davis concerning hereditary deafness in that breed. This research resulted in the BAER test, which became an established part of breeding programs around the country. Two of Dr. Nelson's other projects involved high uric acid in Dalmatians and immune-associated allergies. Dr. Nelson bred Dalmatians under the Forrest prefix, competing in Obedience and conformation for many years. She died prematurely in 1990.

NICHOLAS, ANNA KATHERINE. Born near Troy, New York, Anna Katherine Nicholas owned various dogs through her early years. She received her first dog, a Pekingese, at age seven. Her interest never was in exhibiting but in writing about dogs and then judging.

Her first published article came in the 1930s, and she has continued to write and publish for many dog-related magazines. Her first book, *The Pekingese,* was also published during the 1930s. Since then she has written more than seventy books, including *The Nicholas Guide to Dog Judging* (New York: Howell Book House, 1970), which won the Dog Writers' Association of America award for Best Technical book in 1970.

Anna Katherine judged her first show in 1934 in Hartford, Connecticut. She is approved to judge all Hounds, Terriers, Toys and Non-Sporting breeds plus many of the Sporting dogs, Boxers and Doberman Pinschers. She judged Best in Show at Westminster in 1970, where she has been on the panel eighteen times.

She twice won Gaines FIDO award for Dog Writer of the Year. She received a similar award from *Kennel Review,* and in 1996 she was honored by Heinz pet foods as an inductee into their Hall of Fame.

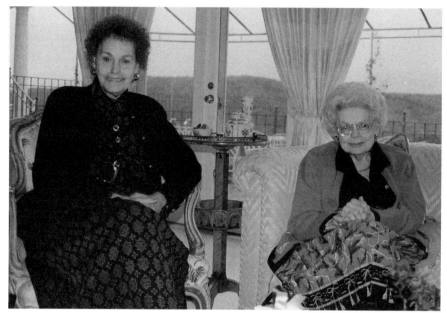

Anna Katherine Nicholas (right), prolific writer, judge and traveler. She is the partner of Marcia Foy (left), whose biography appears in an earlier chapter.

Nicholas has been an officer of many all-breed and National Specialty clubs. She and her partner, Marcia Foy, have lived together for about twenty-five years. At the present time they have two Beagles and two Miniature Poodles that travel by car with them to all the many shows they attend.

NICKLES, DOROTHY D. Dorothy Nickles, a retired high school principal, is an AKC and FCI all-breed judge. She is also approved for all Obedience classes, including Tracking.

Nickles was a breeder of Poodles and Boxers and has shown with great success in both conformation and Obedience in the United States, Canada and Mexico. She is one of the few who won Highest Scoring Dog in Obedience and Best in Show with the same dog (her Standard Poodle) at the same show.

Nickles began to judge in 1952 and after retiring from the educational field has devoted herself full-time to judging throughout the world. She has written articles for magazines and newspapers. She is a popular speaker at clubs and seminars and gives her time to charitable shows and organizations.

An active board member of the Fort Worth Kennel Club, Nickles taught Obedience and Tracking classes for eighteen years and later was made an honorary member of the Tri-City Obedience Club.

In 1988 she was awarded honors as Judge of the Year, and in 1994 she received a Gaines FIDO for Woman of the Year. She was also "roasted" by her friends in Houston, Texas, in conjunction with the Astro World Series of Dog Shows, one of her most memorable experiences.

Dorothy Nickles finds judging a pleasure, a challenge and most rewarding. When not traveling, she calls Fort Worth, Texas, home.

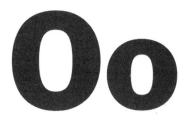

ODUM, W. HENRY III. A dedicated owner and co-owner of several top Brussels Griffons and Border Terriers, Odum started in dogs with a Basset Hound. He is the delegate to the AKC from the American Brussels Griffon Association, and he is the show chairman for Old Dominion Kennel Club, one of the largest outdoor shows in the East.

OLIN, JOHN M. Known for his excellent dogs and success in Field Trials with Labrador Retrievers, John Olin was a major benefactor of veterinary research at Cornell University. In 1950 after losing valuable animals to distemper, he was the force behind the establishment of the Baker Institute for Animal Health. He provided the funds for research into viral diseases, leading to a vaccine against distemper.

Olin is also credited with the establishment of the Orthopedic Foundation for Animals (OFA).

John Olin was the president of Olin, Mathieson, maker of firearms and an avid sportsman. His Nilo kennels produced some of the top Labrador Retrievers in the United States. He also raised Pointers, English Springer Spaniels and Brittanys.

OLSON, PATRICIA, DVM, PhD. Dr. Patricia Olson joined the American Humane Association (AHA) in 1995 as director, Veterinary Affairs and Studies. Before her appointment, Dr. Olson served as a member and chair of AHA's Scientific Advisory Committee and as a member of its board of directors.

Considered a distinguished member of the veterinary profession, Dr. Olson is a member of the National Academies of Practice, where she was chosen by her peers as a person who has made significant and enduring contributions to the practice of veterinary medicine. She received her doctor of veterinary medicine and master of science degrees from the University of Minnesota, as well as a doctorate in reproductive physiology and endocrinology from Colorado State. She has also completed graduate work in biomedical ethics. As a tenured faculty member and instructor, Dr. Olson taught at Cornell University College of Veterinary Medicine, Colorado State University and the University of Minnesota.

She is particularly interested in small animal reproduction and pet overpopulation and is a founding member of the National Council on Pet

Population Study and Policy. In addition, she is interested in issues relating to the use of animals in teaching and biomedical research; the use of genetic engineering; the relationship between abuse to animals and children; production medicine involving food animals and public policies that affect animals.

In 1996, Dr. Olson was awarded the Geraldine R. Dodge Humane Ethics in Action Award, which is given to one humane leader each year in the United States for working to advance the possibilities for a more humane society that treats all forms of life with regard and respect. Also in 1996, she received the American Animal Hospital Association's first-ever Humane Ethics and Animal Welfare Award for her work in advancing animal welfare through extraordinary service and by furthering humane principles, education and understanding.

In 1993 and 1994 Dr. Olson served as a congressional science fellow and professional staff member for the U.S. Senate committee chaired by Senator John D. Rockefeller IV. She authored legislation that was passed and signed into law for research to investigate the causes of Gulf War illnesses in veterans and the association between military exposure and birth defects in offspring. She also served on the staff of several congressional hearings and served as a scientific consultant to numerous senators and staff members.

She has given more than 100 lectures to professional veterinarians and scientists in the United States and seven foreign countries. Much of her academic research focused on the development of nonsurgical methods to prevent pregnancy in animals.

O'NEAL, THOMAS. Dream Ridge Cocker Spaniels and Cavalier King Charles Spaniels have been among the top winning and top producing dogs in those breeds.

Tom O'Neal started with Cockers when he was a student at the University of Wisconsin. Since that time his dogs have been consistent winners in the parti-color variety.

O'NEILL, CHARLES, A. T. and MARI-BETH. "Chuck" O'Neill served as executive vice-president of the American Kennel Club from 1978 until his retirement from that post in the mid-1980s. He was the show chairman for the AKC's Centennial Show, held in Philadelphia in 1984.

O'Neill was an alumnus of the University of Pennsylvania and its Wharton School of Business. He was president and chairman of several refrigerated storage businesses.

He and his family raised Doberman Pinschers, Whippets and Manchester Terriers. He served in many roles in the sport, including show chairman of both Bryn Mawr Kennel Club and the Quaker City Doberman Pinscher Club and the Doberman Pinscher Club of America, for which he was a delegate.

Charles O'Neill died in January 1994.

Mr. O'Neill's daughter, Mari-Beth, was a junior handler of the family's Manchester Terriers. She is now employed by the American Kennel Club as director of the Judge's Education Department. She is also involved with the establishment of an organization for junior handlers through the AKC.

ONOFRIO, JACK. Born on May 11, 1925, in New Haven, Connecticut, Jack Onofrio attended Hill House High School, graduating in June 1942. He entered the U.S. Air Force in November 1942 and served until retirement in August 1965, a career that included action in World War II, Korea and Vietnam.

He attended his first dog show in 1956 and became a licensed all-breed handler in 1962. In 1968 he became a licensed dog show superintendent by buying the MacIver dog show organization. Thus was born Jack Onofrio Dog Shows.

By carefully controlling growth, Jack has expanded the organization from initially running twenty-two shows in 1968 to more than 350 shows in 1996. Jack retired from actively running the organization in 1990, a job that was taken by his son, Jack David, currently chairman and CEO.

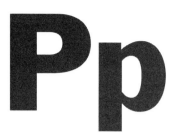

PATTERSON, DONALD F., DVM. Dr. Patterson was born in Venezuela in 1931 and is a graduate of Oklahoma State University, where he received his degree in veterinary medicine in 1954 and was elected to Phi Beta Kappa, a national honors society. In 1956 he entered the U.S. Air Force, where he achieved the rank of captain. He was chief of Laboratory Services at the U.S. Air Force Missile Development Center at Holloman Air Force Base in New Mexico. He served in the air force for two years and upon his return continued his graduate studies in cardiology at the University of Pennsylvania School of Medicine. From 1964 to 1966 he was a Graduate Fellow in Medical Genetics at Johns Hopkins University School of Medicine in Baltimore and in 1967 received his doctor of science in comparative medical sciences at the University of Pennsylvania. Concurrently he did a postgraduate internship at Angell Memorial Animal Hospital in Boston, Massachusetts.

Dr. Patterson was an Instructor in Small Animal Medicine and Surgery at Oklahoma State University School of Veterinary Medicine before going to the University of Pennsylvania, which has been his professional home ever since.

In 1970 he became chief of the first Section of Medical Genetics to be established in a school of veterinary medicine. He initiated the first genetics clinic for animals and the first course in medical genetics for veterinary students. During this period the School of Medicine at the University of Pennsylvania established a Department of Human Genetics, to which Dr. Patterson was appointed and where he is presently a professor of human genetics.

Realizing that research in canine genetics was the key to progress in understanding and controlling genetic defects in dogs and that funds were not generally available for this purpose, in 1974 Dr. Patterson obtained support from the National Institutes of Health for a number of research projects, including studies of the genetics of congenital heart disease, metabolic defects and other genetic disorders in dogs.

His Section of Medical Genetics was the first to standardize dog chromosomes and to detect chromosome defects in dogs. He and his colleagues conducted the first systematic study of inherited metabolic

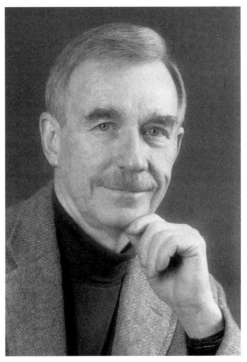

Donald Patterson, DVM, Director of the Center for
Comparative Medical Genetics at the University of
Pennsylvania School of Veterinary Medicine.

defects in dogs and developed some of the first biochemical and molecular
tests for canine genetic disease diagnosis and carrier detection.

In 1994 Dr. Patterson established the Center for Comparative Medical
Genetics at the University of Pennsylvania School of Veterinary Medicine,
an interdepartmental center for the study of genetic diseases in animals.

Dr. Patterson and his colleagues have published more than 200 scientific articles dealing with various aspects of genetic diseases in dogs and in
other animals. In 1989 and 1994 he received National Institutes of Health
Merit awards for his research on canine congenital heart disease, and in
1996 he was chosen by the American Veterinary Medical Association to
receive the American Kennel Club Career Achievement Award in Canine
Research.

Dr. Patterson has developed a comprehensive information database
and resource on genetic diseases in dogs. It will be published in computer
software and book form by 1998 and contain information useful to

breeders and veterinarians for accurate diagnosis and control of more than 350 genetic diseases in more than 200 breeds of dogs existing around the world.

Don Patterson is a member of several professional organizations, is a diplomate of the American College of Veterinary Internal Medicine and is board certified in internal medicine and cardiology.

He is married to Moyra Smith and lives in Wallingford, Pennsylvania.

PEACOCK, SAMUEL M., M.D. Dr. Peacock is a graduate of Princeton University and the School of Medicine of the University of Pennsylvania. He has been on the medical faculty of Tulane University in New Orleans, the University of Pennsylvania in Philadelphia, and Thomas Jefferson University Medical School, also in Philadelphia. He served as a captain in the U.S. Army Medical Corps, assigned to the neuropharmacology branch of the U.S. Army Chemical Center in Edgewood, Maryland. His primary interest is in neurophysiology research with clinical involvement in electroencephalography and sleep medicine. Currently he is a consultant to several sleep disorder laboratories in the Philadelphia area.

Peacock acquired his first two Standard Poodles in 1954 and finished one of them owner-handled in eleven shows. His first litter was whelped in 1957, from which he finished two champions and pointed several others. The Peacocks have campaigned three Specials for multiple–Best in Show wins each and have finished a total of twenty-six Davaroc champions, several of them being top producers.

Dr. Peacock was a charter member of the Creole Poodle Club of New Orleans, has been a board member of the Poodle Club of America for twenty years, serving as president and currently as delegate to the American Kennel Club. He is also a member of the William Penn Poodle Club, the Bryn Mawr Kennel Club, Chester Valley Kennel Club and the Kennel Club of Philadelphia. He has been actively judging since 1973 and has judged the Poodle Club of America National Specialty on several occasions as well as PCA regional and affiliate club Specialties.

In addition to the Poodles, he and his wife, Mary, enjoy landscaping and gardening, especially rhododendrons, daylillies and daffodils, as well as camellias and orchids under glass at their home in Chester Springs, Pennsylvania.

PEPPER, JEFFREY. Jeff Pepper's Pepperhill Kennels started in the late 1960s with a Golden Retriever dog that was purchased as a pet. Competing in Obedience the Peppers were persuaded to try the dog in conformation;

147

this became their introduction to the world of shows. Their foundation bitch was a sister to the great Ch. Cummings Gold-Rush Charlie, and she became a great producer in her own right.

In the 1980s the Peppers added Petit Basset Griffon Vendeen to their Golden household. Jeff is now a licensed AKC judge of many Sporting breeds. He is also on the board of directors of Take the Lead, and he is treasurer of the Dog Judges Association.

PETERS, PATRICIA. A breeder of Lakeland Terriers, Patricia Peters produced one of the top winning and top producing bitches in the history of the breed. Ch. Kilfel Pointe of Vu, "Flirt" won four national Specialties and multiple Bests in Show over a three-year period. She also produced nine champion offspring. In her last appearance at Montgomery County Kennel Club show in 1990 she won the breed from the Veterans class and took third in the Group. During this time she also placed at Westminster. Her sons and daughters have also produced many champion offspring, carrying on the Kilfel line.

PFERD, WILLIAM III. Bill Pferd was born in Elizabeth, New Jersey, in 1922. After receiving graduate degrees in science and engineering he spent the major portion of his career in industrial laboratories, developing communication products.

His broad interest in the physical aspects of history began during a visit to the Roman ruins while serving in Italy as an air force intelligence officer during World War II. His career was paralleled by interests in art and literature.

Bill Pferd and his wife, Jane, bought their first Welsh Springer Spaniel as a family companion in the 1960s. In natural progression, enchanted with their first puppy, they went from one dog to two and then to trainer, handler, breeder and organizer of the breed club of which he became vice-president. Under the Deckard prefix they bred several champions, combining both English and American-bred stock.

Pferd realized that there was no comprehensive literature about this ancient breed, and he spent several years researching the history in the United States and Great Britain. In 1977 *The Welsh Springer Spaniel, History, Selection, Training and Care* (New York: A.S. Barnes, 1977) was published. It has remained as the most important source of information about the breed.

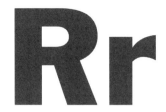

RAYNE, DEREK GLENON. Derek Rayne was born at Raynes Park, Surrey, England, and was educated at Kings College. He showed his first dog, an Airedale Terrier, at age eight. Since then he has owned seventeen different breeds but is best known for his Smooth and Wire Fox Terriers and Pembroke Welsh Corgis. He has been a prominent Corgi breeder for more than fifty years and has campaigned such well-known dogs as English and American Ch. Rockrose of Wey, Ch. Nebriowa Miss Bobbisox and Ch. Elskling of Foxlore, winners of many Specialties and all-breed Bests in Show. Miss Bobbisox won the Working Group at Westminster in 1972.

Mr. Rayne started judging in the United States in 1939. He has been approved for all breeds since 1950 and was, at one time, the youngest all-breed judge in the world, as well as being licensed to judge Obedience Trials.

His overseas assignments have included shows in the British Isles, Australia, New Zealand, Tasmania, Cuba, Mexico, Sweden, Canada, Japan, South Africa, Denmark, Venezuela, Argentina, Brazil and Germany.

Among his most memorable judging assignments have been the Melbourne Royal in 1962, where he judged 3,600 dogs in 9 days, the Blackpool Championship Show in England in 1971, where he judged only the 6 Variety Groups and Best in Show. He judged Best in Show at Westminster in 1983. Mr. Rayne resides in Carmel by the Sea, California, with his wife, the former Gerda Kennedy. Dr. Kennedy is a former physician who came to the United States from Austria. She was a breeder of Afghan Hounds, beginning in 1961. At her home in Oklahoma she also raised Lippizaner horses. She has judged since 1969 and is approved for all Hound breeds and several breeds in the Sporting Group.

Rayne's family owned and operated Derek Rayne, Ltd., a clothing business for men and women for fifty-three years until he retired in 1995. He is an active member of both Santa Barbara and Del Monte Kennel Clubs and is the only living charter member of the latter. He is currently the honorary president of both and is a member of the Kennel Club of England. He won the Gaines FIDO award for Dog Judge of the Year in 1956 and in 1975 won the *Kennel Review* award as Outstanding Judge of the Year. In a 1988 poll conducted by the publication *Canine Chronicle* he was voted number one judge in every Variety Group.

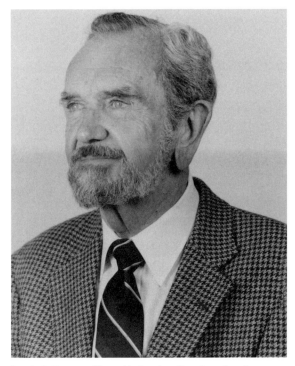

Derek G. Rayne, all-breed judge, longtime breeder of Pembroke Welsh Corgis.

REESE, GLORIA N. Gloria Reese has been involved in the sport of pure-bred dogs since 1953 when her first litter of Collies was born. She began to show in earnest when she and her husband, Nat, bought their first Borzoi. They raised and bred Borzoi for more than twenty-six years, but in 1972 they acquired and campaigned the top winning Doberman Pinscher bitch, Ch. Galaxy's Cory Missile Belle. They won the Working Group at Westminster and the top dog award for 1973. In 1975 they purchased the Greyhound, Ch. Aroi Talk of the Blues. "Punky" became top dog in 1976 and won two Group firsts at Westminster. Their last important campaigner was a Bouvier des Flandres, Ch. Galbraith's Iron Eyes, another Westminster Group winner. Throughout their years of exhibiting top dogs, professional handler Corky Vroom presented their standard-bearers. They are now retired from that aspect of the sport.

Gloria and Nat Reese were both born and raised in Chicago but have lived all their married lives near Los Angeles. They are the parents of three children and grandparents of six.

They are directors of Cedars of Sinai, have donated the Nuclear Research Building for the City of Hope Hospital in Los Angeles and are directors of the Scripps Clinic in La Jolla. They are also major supporters of Morris Animal Foundation.

Gloria is approved to judge all Hound breeds, Pointers, Irish Setters and Doberman Pinschers. She judged the Hound Group at Westminster in 1997.

REMER, MARY. Mary Remer has been actively involved with Bull Terriers for twenty years. Winkie Mackay-Smith of Banbury fame was her mentor and inspiration and has co-bred many dogs with her. Remer's dogs, which bear both Banbury and her kennel name, Bedrock, are among the top dogs in the breed.

Mary Remer strives to maintain breed type while producing dogs that are sound, healthy and able to compete in Obedience and Agility Trials while shining in the conformation ring.

She is cofounder of the Obedience Committee for the Bull Terrier Club of America. She does behavioral evaluations and consultations for Bull Terriers, including many welfare dogs. Her approach to behavioral issues is from a holistic point of view.

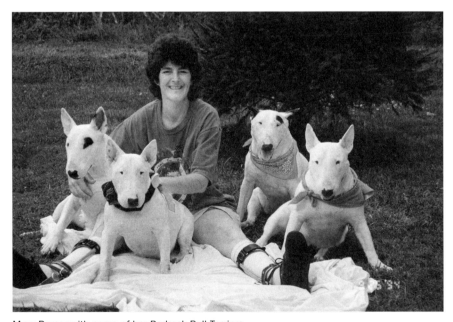

Mary Remer with some of her Bedrock Bull Terriers.

Remer owns her own business that addresses the community and responsible pet ownership. She works with dogs and their owners to find and reinforce the bond that is possible between all dogs and their owners.

RIDDLE, MAXWELL. Considered to be one of the preeminent figures in purebred dogs, Max Riddle is a retired newspaperman and an internationally acclaimed dog writer. He was an all-breed judge and the guiding force behind Ravenna Kennel Club's purchase of its own show site. The cluster of shows at that eastern Ohio location in August has become one of the largest in the country.

He started his career in shows at age fourteen, when he put on his own dog show in Ravenna, Ohio. Although he bred and exhibited American Foxhounds and Great Danes, it was as a prolific writer of dog books, including major sections of the *International Encyclopedia of Dogs* (New York: Howell Book House, 1971) that Riddle is best known. He has won

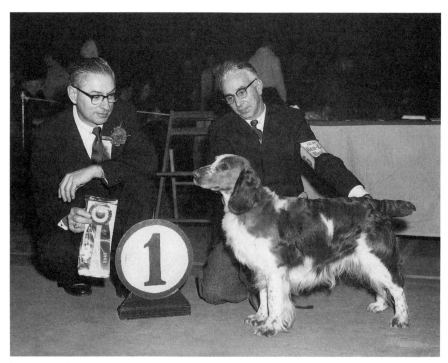

Maxwell Riddle, newspaperman, sportsman and veteran all-breed judge. He is shown here presenting an award to a Welsh Springer Spaniel, handled by D. Lawrence Carswell, whose biography is given in a earlier chapter.

every award offered by the Dog Writers' Association of America, and that group now offers the "Maxwell" awards, named in his honor, for first place in every category of its annual competition. He also won a Gaines FIDO award for Dog Writer of the Year. He was a syndicated columnist with a weekly newspaper column on dogs and other animals, and he wrote extensively for canine publications.

Max Riddle's wife, Leonora is a well-traveled judge and writer in her own right.

RIGDEN, ELAINE. "Lainey" Rigden grew up in a family that raised Chow Chows and Scottish Terriers. She and her late husband, Jerry, were professional handlers starting in 1954, and they also bred Dachshunds, Pembroke Welsh Corgis and Whippets. She also raised Pekingese and is a two-time winner of the Quaker Oats award for Toy Dog of the Year.

Elaine Rigden writes for the canine weekly *Dog News* and is an approved judge of all breeds in the Hound, Terrier, Toy and Non-Sporting Groups.

ROBERTS, PERCY. Born in Great Britain in 1889, Percy Roberts emigrated to the United States in 1913 at the suggestion of J. J. Holgate, a famous English breeder and exporter of dogs. Roberts worked first for Vickery Kennels in Illinois, a large establishment housing many breeds. In 1919 he opened his own kennel, calling it "Revelry." Here he bred Whippets and Greyhounds, but it was as a professional handler and an importer that he made his most enduring mark. He had a talent for recognizing breed type and quality in any dog and was soon buying some of the top dogs in England for his clients in the states.

Among his most famous imports were three Wire Fox Terriers that he selected for the Halleston Kennels of Stanley J. Halle. All three became Best in Show winners at Westminster in 1926, 1934 and 1937. Roberts won a fourth Best in Show there, with a Sealyham Terrier, giving him the record for the most Westminster Bests.

Roberts was associated with the top kennels of the day for decades, including Mr. and Mrs. James Farrell's Foxden kennels, the Mardormere Greyhounds and Whippets of Mr. and Mrs. George Anderson and several others in a variety of breeds. Percy Roberts showed them all.

From 1937 to 1950 Roberts was an enormously successful professional. He retired from that aspect of the sport and almost immediately became an all-breed judge. He judged every major show in the United States and many engagements at Westminster, including the coveted Best in Show assignment in 1967. He judged the Sidney Royal in Australia five times and

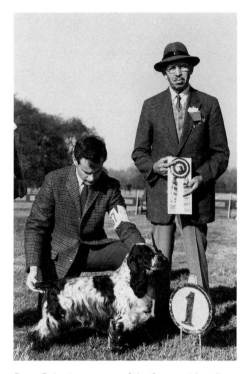

Percy Roberts was one of the foremost handlers of his day and took on the same status as an all-breed judge. He is shown awarding a Specialty Best of Breed to the English Cocker Spaniel, Ch. Dunelm Galaxy, handled by Richard Bauer, whose biography is given in an earlier chapter.

presided at shows in England, South America, Canada, New Zealand and Tasmania. Percy Roberts, considered by those who knew him to be one of the greatest figures in the dog sport, died in 1977.

ROBSON, ISABEL. A longtime breeder and exhibitor of dogs and horses, Robson started early. At age ten she showed her English Setter at the legendary Morris & Essex show. She is best known for her Dalmatians, although she has owned many other breeds, including Pugs, Whippets, Dachshunds and Pembroke Welsh Corgis. Her only Basset Hound, Ch. Slippery Hill Hudson, was the top winning specimen in the breed for many years. She was the co-owner of the 1986 Westminster Best in Show winner,

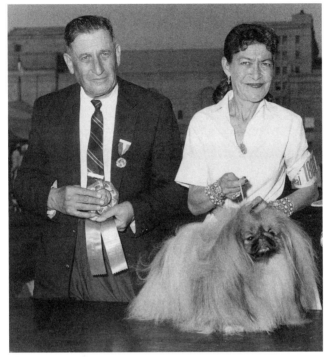

Alva Rosenberg, to many the greatest dog judge of all time, with two other legendary figures, the Pekingese Ch. Chik T'Sun of Caversham and his handler Clara Alford.

a Pointer, Ch. Marjetta's National Acclaim. In 1997 she had two Group winners at Westminster, a Dalmatian, Ch. Spotlight's Spectacular and a Dachshund, Ch. Starbarrack Malachite, SW.

Isabel Robson and her husband, Alan, are major supporters of the University of Pennsylvania School of Veterinary Medicine. They live in Glenmoore, Pennsylvania.

ROSENBERG, ALVA. One of the most influential and respected judges of the early decades of the twentieth century, Alva Rosenberg attended his first dog show, Westminster, when he was eight years old. Fascinated by the atmosphere, he was quickly caught up with what was to become a lifelong passion.

His first dog was a Russian Wolfhound, a gift at age sixteen. He started to show in 1915 with a Boston Terrier, and over the years he bred many good Bostons under his Ravenroyd prefix.

155

Rosenberg's mark was to be made as a judge. In 1910 at age eighteen he judged his first show, and in a career that spanned seven decades he judged all over the United States and in many foreign countries.

He was an antique dealer by profession, first in New York City and later in Wilton, Connecticut. He traveled as often in pursuit of antiques for his clients or his shops as he did for his judging assignments.

In 1946 Rosenberg was chosen *Kennel Review*'s Dog Man of the Year, an honor that was repeated in 1947 and 1948. These three FIDO awards were joined in 1973 by one honoring him as Dog Man of the Year.

Alva Rosenberg died just after that ceremony in March 1973 at age eighty.

ROTH, ANN. Ann Roth was instrumental in establishing the English Foxhound and its foundation stock as show dogs in the United States. Hartnett English Foxhounds appear in the pedigrees of every show kennel in this country today. She imported two hounds from Australia that were crossed with her foundation line, providing the beginnings of several fledgling kennels. She has produced more than 100 champions, including 3 Best in Show winners and innumerable Group winners and placers. Hartnett Hounds were the first to obtain Obedience, Tracking and international championship titles.

Roth is president of the English Foxhound Club of America, which has recently been sanctioned by the American Kennel Club. Her goal is to promote the breed at AKC events, to improve and expand its limited gene pool and to build the national club to further those goals.

Hartnett Hounds are located in Wilmington, North Carolina.

ROTHROCK, MILDRED E. "MID". Mid Rothrock grew up in Washington, D.C., and in Rhode Island. She is a graduate of Mills College with a bachelor of arts. Following a year working at CBS in New York she joined the American Red Cross, serving two and a half years in London and on the continent during World War II. She was married in Paris just before VE day to Major H. D. Rothrock (later lieutenant colonel). The couple moved to California, first to San Francisco and then to Marin County and Sonoma County. Rothrock currently lives in Sebastopol, California.

The couple acquired their first Rottweiler in 1953 and became involved in conformation and Obedience, earning eighteen Obedience titles and two championships. Mid currently owns two Rottweilers, a Champion, UDT male and a young CD bitch, as well as a CDX, TD Papillon. Mid became a Tracking judge in 1972 and later was approved to judge all Obedience classes and TDX tests.

One Rottweiler bitch earned a Herding title from the American Herding Breeds Association. Enthusiasm for this activity led her to serve on the American Rottweiler Club Herding Committee, which successfully petitioned the AKC to admit Rottweilers to AKC Herding tests.

A retired executive and school district secretary, Mid Rothrock has served in many volunteer capacities. Her memberships include the Marin County Dog Training Club, American Rottweiler Club, Western Rottweiler Owners, Papillon Club of America, Senior Conformation Judges Association, American Dog Show Judges Association and Northern California Obedience Judges Association.

She has judged throughout the continental United States, Hawaii and Alaska.

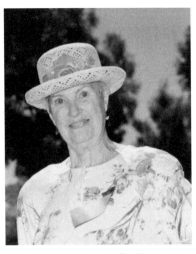

Mildred "Mid" Rothrock, Obedience and Tracking judge, breeder of Rottweilers.

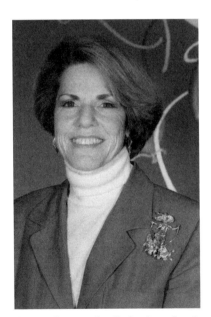

Eleanor Rotman, Poodle fancier, adjunct college professor, judge of conformation and Obedience.

ROTMAN, ELEANOR. Ellie Rotman grew up with Pomeranians in New York City. After completing her education she received a gift of a Miniature Poodle and in 1966 began obedience training. She showed her dog in Obedience and conformation, and since then has bred and owned both Miniature and Standard varieties. Some of her dogs have accomplished their Obedience titles and breed championships at the same time.

Rotman began judging Obedience in 1970 and conformation in 1979. She is currently approved to judge all Non-Sporting and Toy breeds, most of the Sporting Group and all Obedience classes. She has judged at all the major shows within the United States, as well as in Canada, Bermuda, Puerto Rico, Hawaii, Australia, Taiwan, England, South America and Ireland.

Rotman has been president, show chairman and headed various committees for the Ramapo Kennel Club. She has also been president and held many other positions for the Watchung Mountain Poodle Club. She was a delegate to the American Kennel Club for twelve years and was a member of two advisory committees during that time. As a member of the Association of Obedience Clubs and Judges, she served as chairman of the D'Ambrisi award. For the past twelve years she has organized and chaired the Tri-State Dog Judges Workshop, and is on the board of directors of the American Dog Show Judges Association.

Ellie Rotman is a school psychologist, an adjunct college professor and wife of a practicing clinical psychologist. She is proud of her son and daughter-in-law, who have two dogs. She has been active in professional organizations, both on the local and national levels, and her credentials are listed in *Who's Who in American Women*.

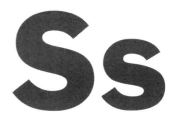

SABELLA, FRANK. A native New Yorker, Frank Sabella had always wanted a dog but never was allowed to have one. When he moved into his own apartment in 1955, he immediately bought a Standard Poodle through an ad in the *New York Times.* That was the beginning of his association with purebred dogs. He began to show his bitch, but at his first show he spotted a young woman handling and took his bitch to her. She finished easily, but more important, that chance meeting was the beginning of a long association with Anne Rogers Clark.

Sabella's varied career began in show business, where he was a dancer with the New York City Ballet and subsequently went on tour with his own dance group. After a move to California to continue his career, he grew tired of traveling and looked for another avenue for his talents. Through his Poodles he met Ann and Tom Stevenson, important breeders and exhibitors who encouraged him to become a professional handler. In 1960 he became associated with his first important client, and from that time until 1974 when he applied for judging approval, he handled some of America's top dogs. He was associated primarily with Poodles and other coated breeds because his clients recognized his talent and ability to present them to their best advantage.

Perhaps Frank Sabella's most successful charge was the white Standard Poodle, Ch. Acadia Command Performance who culminated a brilliant show career with the coveted Best in Show honors at Westminster in 1973.

Sabella's talent with design and flowers is well known in the dog Fancy. He has owned floral establishments and has dressed some of the finest banquets and social occasions in the dog world.

He is the author of two books and numerous articles for the dog press.

He was the recipient of the *Kennel Review*'s Top Male Handler award and was awarded a Gaines FIDO for Dog Man of the Year.

Frank Sabella has approval to judge all Toy and Non-Sporting breeds, most of the Sporting and Hound Groups, plus some Terriers and part of the Working Group. He has judged championship events in Australia, Brazil, England, Scandinavia, four times in Japan and has judged eight times at Westminster, including the exalted Best in Show assignment in 1990. He lives in Treasure Island, Florida.

SACKS, RITA L. Pharaoh Hounds and Rita Sacks are synonymous, although the rare breed was not her first experience with purebred dogs. Rita grew up in Brooklyn, New York, and was a student of piano before deciding that being a concert pianist was not her true calling. She changed her focus and went to New York University to study art and English.

She and her husband at that time bought a Doberman Pinscher that she bred and then added a few Rottweilers until she saw a picture of a Pharaoh Hound. Sachs decided that would be her breed, and for two years she researched the breed in depth and tried to find a puppy. In 1969 her determination paid off, and she acquired her first Pharaoh Hound.

The following year she and a small group of breeders founded the Pharaoh Hound Club of America (PHCA), and Sachs became the registrar of the Stud Book. From 1970 to 1995 she published and edited their newsletter, *Hieroglyphics*. She has been the breed columnist for the *AKC Gazette* since the breed was admitted to the Hound Group in 1984. She has served as secretary of the club since its inception, and she coauthored a book on the breed, *The Pharaoh Hound* (Fairfax, Virginia: Denlinger Alpine, 1983). She is also the Judges Education Committee coordinator and helped produce the PHCA's illustrated Standard for the breed.

She credits her daughter, Laurie Laventhall, for much of the work done on the registry and stud book. She is also cobreeder on most of the champions bred under their kennel name, Beltara.

SAKAYEDA, FRANK. Frank Sakayeda began to import, sell and breed Shiba Inus in the United States in 1978. His frequent trips to Japan continue to enable him to see some of the top dogs in the breed's native country. Before AKC recognition, dogs of his breeding were quietly distributed throughout the United States, and their names can be found in a great number of Shiba pedigrees today.

He imported and co-owned Ch. Toyojiro of Nidaimanei Sow, ROM, the top winning Shiba for 1993 and 1994. That dog sired Ch. San Jo Wise Guy, also co-owned by Sakayeda. Wise Guy was the top Shiba for 1995.

Through his program of buying and breeding top imports, he is currently the strongest influence on the Shiba breed.

SAUNDERS, BLANCHE. One of the pioneers of dog training and Obedience, Blanche Saunders's book, *Training You to Train Your Dog,* became the bible of those who aspired to teach Obedience and those who tried to learn.

The daughter of a Baptist minister and a graduate of Massachusetts State College, she taught Obedience to dogs and students from 1934 until her death in 1968. She became a teacher of teachers and conducted special courses and clinics for Obedience instructors, the first person in the field to do so. She was the first instructor to attempt to popularize Obedience for the average pet owner, demonstrating how a simple course of Obedience exercises could make an out-of-control animal into an enjoyable companion.

SAVORY, ANNE D. Presently the director of AKC's field staff, Anne Savory's background is in dogs. She and her former husband, Dr. John Savory, both of whom came from England in 1961, started Dunholm Irish Setters in 1963 with a bitch from Tirvelda Kennels of E. I. Eldredge. They had great success with their dogs, finishing thirty-five champions, including one that went on to become a Best in Show winner. Savory became a professional handler in 1970 first on her own and then in partnership with Bill Pace, building a training center and boarding facility.

She started her career with the AKC as a field representative working in the southwest in 1984 and in 1995 was promoted to her present position. When not traveling she enjoys gourmet cooking and gardening. She also enjoys needlework and reading.

SAWYER-BROWN, BARBARA. Barbara Sawyer-Brown has been involved with Rhodesian Ridgebacks since purchasing her first dog in 1966. Since then she has bred seventy champions. She is the only breeder in the United States to have produced five all-breed Best in Show Ridgebacks. Nine of her dogs have ranked in the top ten for the breed, and five of these were number one. Her dogs and bitches have also been top producers and have formed the foundation stock for other breeders.

Her kennel name, Kwetu, a Swahili word meaning "our home," depicts their atmosphere. Her dogs are house pets. She does not have kennels.

Brown is currently approved to judge fourteen breeds in the Hound Group, including Rhodesian Ridgebacks. She has judged the breed twice in Australia, New Zealand and the Rhodesian Ridgeback Club of the United States National Specialty show. In 1995 she judged the breed in Sweden and in 1996 in England, Denmark, Holland and Israel.

She is past president of the Rhodesian Ridgeback Club of the United States and an honorary member of the Rhodesian Ridgeback Club of Western Australia. She is past president of the Carolina Kennel Club and past director of the Nashville Kennel Club. She is associate editor of the *Ridgeback Quarterly* and a published writer of breed-related articles.

Barbara Sawyer-Brown resides in Chicago, Illinois.

SCHULTZ, BRUCE AND GRETCHEN. Bruce and Gretchen Schultz have both been passionately involved in dogs and the sport of dogs their entire lives. Bruce, born and raised in Minnesota, was actively involved in sports and hunting. His hunting dog and companion was a German Shorthaired Pointer. Moving to Phoenix, Arizona, after completing his military service, he purchased an Irish Setter. Becoming involved in Obedience led him into exploring conformation, where he met and hired professional handlers Bob and Patty Grant. After being a client, apprentice and eventually an assistant to the Grants, Bruce ventured out on his own in the early to mid-1970s specializing in setters, breeding English Setters under the Rimrock prefix. He produced numerous champions, Group and Specialty winners.

Gretchen, born and raised in southern California, is the daughter of well-known handlers and breeders, Walt and Joyce Shellenbarger. Breeding German Shorthaired Pointers under the Gretchenhof prefix, they produced a strong foundation for today's Shorthairs and count among many accomplishments the coveted Best in Show award at Westminster in 1974 won with Ch. Gretchenhof Columbia River.

Gretchen Schultz grew up with dogs, traveling and assisting her parents throughout her childhood. After an absence from shows to complete her education and pursue a career, she returned to the show ring, traveling with her mother and showing her own German Shorthaired Pointer. She met Bruce at her first show, and they were married in 1978.

Together Bruce and Gretchen have created a very successful handling team, showing dogs in five Groups, campaigning numerous top winning dogs. Included in their accomplishments are Group wins at Westminster, piloting Quaker Oats awards winners, winning more than 250 Bests in Show and multiple National Specialty wins in a variety of breeds.

With an older ranch home and a kennel situated in an orange grove in Riverside, California, they refer to their operation as "Camp Schultz." They maintain only the dogs that they show for conditioning and training. With clients around the world they have had opportunities to travel to Japan and to Brazil to show dogs for their clients and to judge.

Bruce is an avid fisherman, and both Bruce and Gretchen are enthusiastic golfers. They have two children and two grandchildren. They both enjoy cooking, and when they are not on the road, together they plan and prepare gourmet meals for the family. Bruce and Gretchen are members of PHA and are Certified Professional Handlers.

SCHWARTZ, ALEXANDER AND GLORVINA. Sandy and Glorvina Schwartz are known for their top winning Afghan Hounds and more recently Norwich Terriers that they breed and show under the Sandina prefix.

Glorvina grew up with dogs. Her uncle, Gerald Livingston, was president of Westminster from 1937 to 1942. Her aunt gave Glorvina, as a girl, her first dog, a Labrador Retriever. She was also noted for Miniature Pinschers and Pugs, and Glorvina's first show dogs were Pugs. Glorvina is the handler, Sandy is the judge. Sandy's family were breeders of thoroughbred horses, having won the Kentucky Derby and the Preakness Stakes with a home-bred in 1938. His father's steeplechase horse also won the Grand National at Aintree, England, in 1926.

Sandina Kennels has produced the top Afghan Hound in America with three different dogs, 1975, 1977 and 1979, and in 1980 one of the dogs won the Quaker Oats award for top Hound, bred,

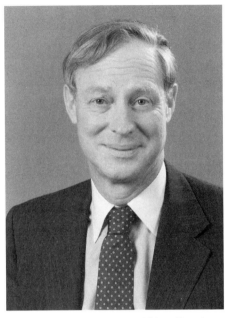

Alexander "Sandy" Schwartz, Afghan Hound and Norwich Terrier breeder, judge and member of Westchester and Westminster Kennel Clubs.

owned and handled by Glorvina. Their Norwich Terriers have won the National Specialty at Montgomery County from 1994 through 1997 and in 1997 the Specialty winner, the year's top show dog, went on to Best in Show.

Sandy has been employed by the Prudential Insurance Company of America as an investment banker for the past thirty-three years.

He is a judge of all Hound, Working, Terrier, Toy and Non-Sporting breeds, having officiated internationally for more than twenty years.

Sandy is president of Tuxedo Park Kennel Club, secretary-treasurer of Westchester Kennel Club, a member of Westminster Kennel Club, Palm Beach County Dog Fanciers Association and the Pug Dog Club of America. The Schwartzs live in Tuxedo Park, New York.

SCULLY, PATRICIA. Pat Scully has been active in purebred dogs since 1962. She has bred and shown Pugs in Obedience and conformation in the United States, Bermuda, Canada and Mexico. She has been an approved Obedience judge for all classes in the United States, Bermuda and Canada for more than twenty-five years.

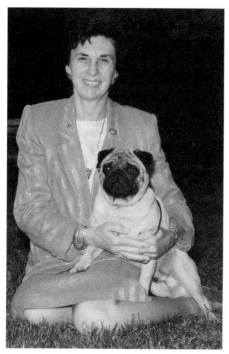

Patricia "Pat" Scully, Obedience judge, Pug breeder and member of the AKC board of directors.

A graduate of Cornell University, she worked until her 1994 retirement as a cardiovascular pharmacologist at Lederle Laboratories in the field of clinical trials for hypertension.

She has held offices in many dog clubs, including past president of the Pug Dog Club of America, Inc., in which she is a lifetime honorary member; former president of the Association of Obedience Clubs and Judges, Inc.; former Obedience chairman, member of the board of directors and honorary lifetime member of Ramapo Kennel Club; honorary lifetime member of the K-9 Obedience Training Club of Essex County, New Jersey; treasurer, Obedience chairman and member of the board of directors of Tuxedo Park Kennel Club. She is delegate to the AKC for the Obedience Training Club of Hawaii, Inc., and in March 1997, she was elected to a four-year term on the board of directors of the AKC.

Scully also rode in horsemanship and junior hunter competition as an equestrian. She resides in Suffern, New York.

SECHER, COLETTE. Now a photojournalist, Colette Secher was born in Algeria and grew up traveling back and forth between France and the United States. After moving to Chicago with her family, Secher acquired her first show dog, an Irish Setter. She became fascinated with the show world and began working as an assistant to the late, great professional handler, Jack Funk. However, she preferred showing her own dogs, and although various business commitments prevented her from keeping many dogs, she always had a few.

In 1978 she married George Secher and began showing Smooth Fox Terriers under the LeFox prefix. Her first encounter with French Bulldogs was in Paris, although she did not buy a dog there, but found her foundation stock in California. She has since owned and bred some of the top French Bulldog studs, as well as six-time Best in Show winner, Ch. LeFox Steel Magnolia.

Mme. Secher lives in Bannock-burn, Illinois.

SECORD, WILLIAM. Bill Secord was the first director of the Dog Museum, now called AKC's Museum of the Dog. Educated in fine arts, he is the curator of several exhibitions on dog art, both in the United States and abroad. After leaving the Dog Museum he opened his own gallery in New York City, specializing in canine art, bronzes and objets d'art. He is the author of two historical retro-spectives on canine art.

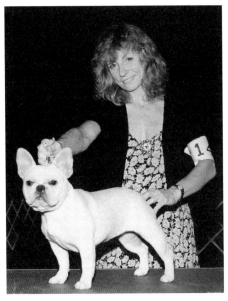

Mme. Colette Secher with one of her LeFox French Bulldogs.

SEELEY, EVA. A large measure of the success of the Siberian Husky and the Alaskan Malamute as purebred sled and show dogs is due to the efforts of this memorable New Englander who went by the nickname "Short" Seeley. In the 1920s the Seeleys took over the Chinook kennels of Arthur Walden, who left to travel with Admiral Byrd. At their home, Wonalancet in New Hampshire, Short and her husband, Milton, established a school for dogs and dog drivers. Dogs that they supplied have served in the armed forces, have gone on Antarctic expeditions and have made history in the sport of dog sledding.

The Seeleys favored Alaskan Malamutes and Siberian Huskies. It was primarily through their efforts that a true, purebred Alaskan Malamute was recognized by the American Kennel Club in 1935. They organized the Alaskan Malamute Club of America and kept the New England Sled Dog Club alive after its first president went to Antarctica.

Short Seeley was one of three women who raced on New England trails in the 1930s. During the almost fifty years that Chinook Kennels was in existence more than 2,000 dogs went through the establishment.

Short was a breeder, judge and honorary life president of the Siberian Husky Club of America. In 1971 her name was read into the Congressional

Record, citing her unique contribution to the world of northern dogs. In 1976 her book, coauthored with Max Riddle, *The Complete Alaskan Malamute* (New York: Howell Book House, 1976), was named best breed book of the year by the Dog Writers' Association of America.

SHAY, SUNNY. From 1947 until her sudden death while in the ring in 1978, Sunny Shay played an important part of the development of the Afghan Hound in the United States. Shay was a star-crossed fancier, outliving disasters, including a fire that gutted her kennel and took the lives of many of her dogs. At that time Sunny moved to the home of Roger Rechler on Long Island, and the remaining dogs became jointly owned as a continuation of her Grandeur Kennels. On the day she died she was handling the latest Grandeur special, Ch. Blu Boy of Grandeur. It was said of Sunny Shay that she went out as she would have wanted to—showing in the ring. After her collapse, Mike Canalizo took the dog and won the Hound Group. The next in line was a Blu Boy son, Ch. Blue Shah of Grandeur, which started Roger Rechler and Mike Canalizo on a winning trajectory carrying forward to the present.

SHELLEY, HELEN. Helen Shelley's first German Wirehaired Pointer was Ch. Mueller Mills Valentino. Handled by Roy Murray, he had a spectacular career, winning the National Specialty in 1963 and seven all-breed Bests in Show. Helen Shelley is also noted for owning top Brittanys. She is a judge of all Sporting breeds and lives in Tucson, Arizona.

SHERLOCK, HELEN "SCOOTIE." Helen Sherlock, who is always known as Scootie, started her life with German Shepherd Dogs by importing her foundation stock, but she has become the voice of the German Shepherd breed in matters of health and longevity. She has been a longtime member of the board of directors of the German Shepherd Dog Club of America, for which she chairs the Genetics Committee. She is also a member of the board of directors of the Orthopedic Foundation for Animals. Scootie lives in Labadie, Missouri.

SIEGAL, MORDECAI. Current president of the Dog Writers Association and a prolific writer, Siegal began his successful writing career with publication of his foremost dog book, *Good Dog, Bad Dog* (1973). This book is still in print, updated in 1991. His second longest–running book is *When Good Dogs Do Bad Things* (1986) and is still relevant as a behavior problem-solving book for dog owners. Altogether he has written twenty-one books.

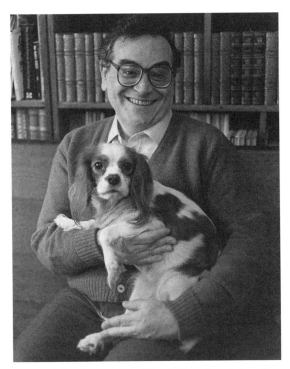

Mordecai Siegal, president of Dog Writers Association of
America with his Cavalier King Charles Spaniel, Philadelphia.

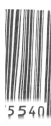
5540

He has written many newspaper and magazine columns, including a long-running feature in *Ladies Home Journal* about dog and cat care, and has published commissioned booklets on the same subjects. He has been a professional communicator, appeared on and in many local TV and radio broadcasts. He has won several awards for his writing, among them Communicator of the Year, 1987, the highest award given annually by the Dog Writers' Association of America, and the Gaines FIDO as Dog Writer of the Year for 1996.

Siegal lives in New York City with his wife and collaborator, Vicky. They have three children and a red tabby cat, Texas. At present they are without a dog, after the death of their Cavalier King Charles Spaniel.

SILLS, NELSON A. A member of the American Kennel Club board of directors from 1980 until 1994, Nelson Sills has been an active participant in Field Trials with his Labrador Retrievers since 1959.

167

He trained and handled the 1964 National Amateur Retriever Champion Dutchmoors Black Mood. He served as president of the National Retriever Club and the Del Bay Retriever Club and is the AKC delegate for the Labrador Retriever Club of America.

Sills graduated from Virginia Polytechnic Institute in 1945, following three years of service in the U.S. Navy in World War II. He did graduate studies at Penn State University, preceding a long career as a civil engineer. He and his wife, Nancy, have four children. They live in Houston, Delaware.

SIMON, MARJORIE. Marjorie Simon has been breeding and showing her Stardust Brussels Griffons since the early 1960s. Ch. Barmere's Mighty Man was the foundation of her early breeding program. She was the founding president of the National Brussels Griffon Club (NBGC) and has served on the boards of both the American Brussels Griffon Association (ABGA) and NBGC for many years. She is currently vice-president of ABGA. She was a member of the Breed Standard Committee and serves on the Illustrated Breed Standard Committee and Judges Education Committee. In 1994 she created the slide presentation for the breed.

Simon founded and directs the Brussels Griffon Rescue operation from her home in Houston, Texas.

SIMONDS, MARSHALL "PETE". Pete Simonds has been a member of the Labrador Retriever Club for thirty years and an active director for the past fifteen years. He also serves as a delegate to the AKC from the Midwest Field Trial Club. He is chairman of the AKC Delegates Committee on Field Trial Clubs, a member of the AKC Northeast Trial Board on disciplinary matters and chairman of the subcommittee on Rules of the Retriever Advisory Committee. Simonds is on the board of directors of the Orthopedic Foundation of America (OFA). He and his wife, Kate, are active in Field Trials and Hunting Tests.

SINKINSON, THE REVEREND, GEORGE, JR., AND JACKIE. The Rectory Bloodhounds began in 1964 with a bitch who turned out to be a good show dog, trailing hound and superior brood bitch. Both George and Jackie grew up in Rhode Island, moved to California and later to Owings Mills, Maryland, where they bred the majority of the more than fifty champions produced at their renowned Rectory Kennel. One of their most famous dogs, Ch. Rectory's Recruit (1965–75) was the top winning Bloodhound in 1969, and he was the sire of twelve champions.

After Reverend Sinkinson's retirement the couple moved to Maine, where they continue to breed dogs for trailing and shows.

SKARDA, LANGDON. A native of New Mexico and a breeder-exhibitor of German Shepherd Dogs, Lang Skarda was a rancher, raising Hereford cattle and goats on a large spread in New Mexico.

In the 1960s he had five Best in Show Shepherds out at the same time. But it was as a judge that Skarda was best known and revered as one of the greats. He started judging in 1947 and became an all-rounder in 1970. His opinions were eagerly sought, and he judged at all the major shows in the United States and in several foreign countries.

Lang Skarda was a wonderful raconteur and could regale a dinner crowd with endless stories and entertainment. He was also a patient teacher and a friend on whom the dog Fancy could depend. Skarda died in March 1994 at age eighty.

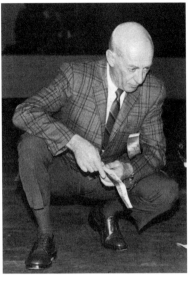

Langdon L. Skarda, German Shepherd Dog breeder and all-breed judge. Judge of Best in Show at Westminster in 1981.

SMITH, C. SEAVER. Considered to be the senior breeder and historian of Great Pyrenees in the United States, Seaver and his wife, Edith, have bred the big white dogs as well as Pembroke Welsh Corgis for more than forty years. Edith owned a Pyr while she was at college in 1945. After she married Seaver they acquired all the best stock owned by Marjorie Butcher.

Their Quibbletown Pyrs were the top winning and top producing dogs in the breed during the 1960s and 1970s. The Smiths finished between 165 and 170 champions. Both were well-respected judges of Working and Herding breeds. Edith passed away in 1989, but Seaver continues to judge. He has been asked to judge the National Specialty for the third time in 1997. Currently, Seaver is concentrating on writing a breed history video from his home in Taunton, Massachusetts.

SMITH, GAIL K., VMD, PhD. Gail Smith received his VMD from the University of Pennsylvania in 1974, completed his orthopedic surgical residency in 1979 and was awarded a PhD in engineering in 1982.

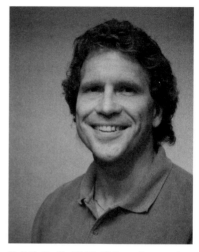

He is currently professor and chief of surgery in the Department of Clinical Studies at the University of Pennsylvania School of Veterinary Medicine. In his research Dr. Smith has applied engineering principles to investigate the canine musculoskeletal system in both health and disease.

Orthopedic problems of the spine, knee and hip are areas of particular interest to him. He has been published more than 100 times on orthopedic topics in the scientific literature.

Gail K. Smith, VMD, PhD, professor of orthopedic surgery and chief of surgery at the University of Pennsylvania School of Veterinary Medicine.

A recent and clinically relevant product of his research is a stress-radiographic diagnostic method capable of predicting the susceptibility to hip dysplasia in dogs as young as sixteen weeks of age. The method, called PennHIP, is now an international program. It holds great promise to reduce the high frequency of canine hip dysplasia by providing improved accuracy in the selection of dogs that are used for breeding.

SMITH, DR. HARRY. In 1957 Dr. Harry Smith and his wife bought their first Pug, Pugholm's Little Jumping Joan. She became the foundation bitch of his kennel. He showed only locally in southern Ohio and northern Kentucky, and he finished several Pug champions with only a limited breeding program.

He was cofounder of the Pug Dog Club of Cincinnati and became its first president in the early 1960s. He owned the first black Pug to win the national futurity.

Dr. Smith was a delegate to the American Kennel Club for the Pug Dog Club of America for ten years and a delegate of the Troy, New York Kennel Club for five years.

He received his first approval to judge in 1966 and since then has been approved for six Groups: Sporting, Working, Terrier, Toy, Non-Sporting and Herding. During thirty years of judging he has judged at Westminster, most of the other major shows in the United States and in several foreign countries. He has been to Sweden, Finland, South Africa and Australia. He is scheduled to return to Sweden and Australia within the next two years.

Dr. Smith received his PhD from North Carolina State University in 1951. In the ensuing years he became an associate director in Industrial Engineering at Proctor & Gamble, dean of the School of Management at RPI in Troy, New York, professor at the University of North Carolina and chairman of the Department of Biomathematical Sciences at the Mount Sinai Medical School in New York City. He has published three books, one of which has been translated into Russian, Polish, French and Spanish. He has also published more than 140 articles in major medical, statistical and mathematical journals.

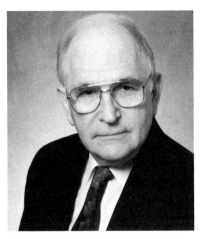

Dr. Harry Smith, retired chairman of the Department of Biomathematical Sciences at Mount Sinai Medical School in New York City. Now a full-time judge of six Groups.

Dr. Smith is now retired and has become a full-time judge. He is also a Life Master Contract Bridge Player and an approved, but inactive, tournament director for the American Contract Bridge League (ACBL).

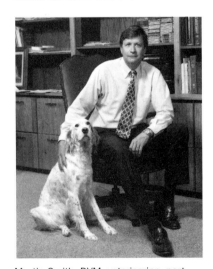

Martin Smith, DVM, veterinarian, part owner of Drs. Foster & Smith, Inc., and pet supply catalog merchandiser.

SMITH, MARTIN, DVM. Dr. Smith graduated from the University of Maryland in 1972 with honors. He then proceeded to receive his DVM in 1976 from Iowa State University. He is a member of the Wisconsin Veterinary Medical Association.

Since graduation he has practiced small animal medicine and surgery and has devoted many hours to wildlife treatment and rehabilitation. He assisted in developing the Northwoods Wildlife Center in 1980, which is still in existence. He is also part owner, with Dr. Race Foster, of one of the largest pet supply mail-order catalog companies, Drs. Foster & Smith, Inc.

With his wife, Kathy, and their five daughters, Dr. Smith enjoys a wide range of activities, including camping, hiking, boating, wildlife photography and skiing. He divides his time between his family, his practice and writing and consulting with other writers, organizations and pet breeders across the United States.

SMITH, DR. ROBERT D. Dr. Smith and his wife, Polly, whom he married in 1959, bred American Foxhounds under the prefix Hazira for more than twenty years. They produced three generations of Best in Show Foxhounds and five generations of Group winning hounds in AKC shows, despite a lack of competition within that breed. They gave up breeding and showing Foxhounds due to the press of business commitments and judging assignments, but Dr. Smith has remained active in the sport for almost forty years.

He was approved to judge his first two breeds, Beagles and American Foxhounds, in 1969 and has gradually added to his roster. In 1996 he was approved to judge all breeds.

Dr. Smith graduated from the University of Virginia with a BA and received a doctorate in political science from Vanderbilt University. He taught at the college and graduate levels for more than ten years. He has twenty-five years of business experience in economic development, including ten years as an industrial developer for Mississippi and fifteen years as a consultant to small and medium-sized business firms.

He semiretired from his profession in 1996 and in that year became a delegate to the AKC from the Huntington Kennel Club. In 1997 he was elected to a four-year term on the AKC's board of directors.

Bob and Polly Smith reside in St. Stephens Church, Virginia.

SOSA, LUIS AND PATRICIA. Bandog French Bulldogs was established in the 1980s after the Sosas had bred and exhibited Bullmastiffs. Since that time the Sosas have bred more than 40 champion Frenchies and have won 13 all-breed Bests in Show, more than 100 Group firsts, hundreds of Bests of Breed and Group placements and 3 National Specialties. Bandog French Bulldogs have been in the top 5 rankings each year since 1989.

Luis and Patricia Sosa are professional photographers and reside in Metairie, Louisiana.

SPADAFORI, GINA. A resident of Sacramento, California, Gina Spadafori is the author of *Dogs for Dummies,* which won the Ralston Purina Award for Excellence from the Dog Writers' Association of America in 1997. Her other writing awards from DWAA include best newspaper column, the

Geraldine R. Dodge award and the outstanding journalist award from Pedigree. She has written a syndicated newspaper column on pets and their care since 1985. She is also on the Internet with a pet-care column.

Spadafori serves on the board of directors of the Dog Writers' Association and the Cat Writers' Association. She shares her home with Andy, a Shetland Sheepdog, and Benjamin, a Flat Coated Retriever.

SPENCER, JAMES. Jim Spencer has been involved in dogs and "dog games" for more than forty years. He has been associated primarily with Golden Retrievers but has also worked with Labrador Retrievers, Chesapeake Bay Retrievers, English Springer Spaniels and Pointers.

He has participated in hunting tests, Field Trials, Obedience Trials and conformation and is a judge of hunting tests for retrievers and spaniels. He bred Golden Retrievers under the prefix Rumrunner but is no longer active in that aspect of the sport.

Spencer has been writing about dogs for sixteen years. He has published five books about training for pointing, flushing and retrieving dogs. He produced a video, and he writes both columns and articles for several outdoor magazines.

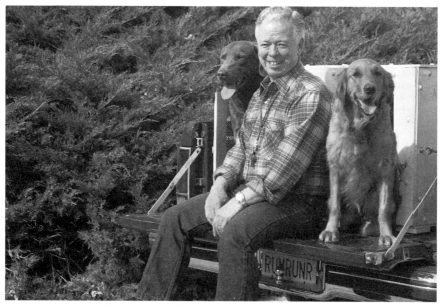

James B. Spencer, Field Trial and hunting enthusiast and writer with two of his Golden Retrievers.

He has been married for forty-two years to Theresa Spencer and has six children and four grandchildren. His education was in business administration for which he received a masters in mathematics. Spencer is a retired systems analyst and EDP auditor. The Spencers call Wichita, Kansas, home.

SPRUNG, DENNIS B. Dennis Sprung exhibited and bred Afghan Hounds and Greyhounds for more than twenty years before joining the staff of the American Kennel Club in 1989. Dogs owned, bred or cobred by him and his wife, Susan, have won more than 150 Bests in Show, as well as the National Specialty in both breeds. He had been approved to judge Afghan Hounds, Greyhounds, Beagles, Whippets, Poodles and Junior Showmanship.

Sprung began his career with AKC as a field representative. In April 1990, he became assistant vice-president of Dog Events and a year later assumed the additional responsibility of director of field staff. In 1993 he was appointed director of Dog Events and in March of 1994 was promoted to

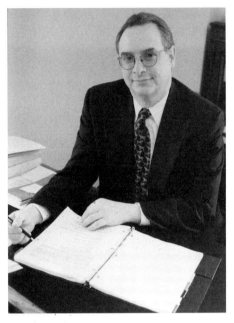

Dennis Sprung, vice-president of Long Range Planning and Development for the American Kennel Club.

vice-president of Show Events. His current position is vice-president for Long Range Planning and Development.

He has served the dog community in many capacities. He was president of the venerable Bronx County Kennel Club from 1978 to 1988 and its AKC delegate for nine years. He was a member of the Delegate Show Operations Committee and an AKC Trial board member. He was on the Planning Committee for the Dog Museum and served as national vice-president of the Owner-Handlers Association, delegate to the New York State Attorney General's Legislative Committee on Animal Care and delegate to the Associated Dog Clubs of New York State.

In 1993 Dennis was awarded the Gaines FIDO for Man of the Year.

The Sprungs reside on Long Island and hold memberships in the Westbury Kennel Association, Bronx County Kennel Club, the Afghan Hound Club of America and the Greyhound Club of America.

STACY, W. TERRY. Terry Stacy was born in Columbus, Ohio, grew up in Pittsburgh, Pennsylvania, and attended Marietta College in Ohio. In 1959 he joined Sears Roebuck in their management training program, and after two years he made up his mind that dogs would be his profession.

Stacy made his debut in the show ring in 1952, handling a Cocker Spaniel in Junior Showmanship. Cockers were his first breed, and he won his first Group with a home-bred Cocker in 1956.

His first job in dogs was as manager of William Brainard's Downsbragh Kennel, gaining experience working with Fox Terriers, Labradors and Greyhounds. He received his handler's license in 1961, one year before he was inducted into the U.S. Army. He served for three years and upon return to civilian life took up his handling career for the next fourteen years. He and his former wife, Charlotte, were known for their presentation of top winning Cockers.

In 1978 Stacy retired from handling and moved to North Carolina to work with the Moss-Bow Dog Show Organization as a superintendent. He left that position in 1981 to join the staff at AKC. He rose to become the AKC's executive vice-president until his retirement in 1995.

Terry Stacy was awarded the Gaines FIDO for Man of the Year in 1995. He and his wife, Jackie, reside in California.

STANDER, MATTHEW H. Matt is a native New York "cityite" who graduated from Columbia College and the University of Virginia Law School. His thirty-six-year career in the sport of purebred dogs has run the gamut from breeder-exhibitor to publisher and editor of major magazines and newspapers devoted to the purebred dog.

His Cragsmoor Kennel prefix has been associated with Bloodhounds, Beagles, Skye Terriers, Airedales, Whippets and most recently English Toy Spaniels.

Stander has twice been awarded the Gaines FIDO for Writer of the Year and once was so honored by *Kennel Review*.

Prior to his professional involvement with the dog world he was real estate house counsel for the American Oil Company, president of Sara Fredericks, Inc., a retail chain, and director of development for the Kenton Corporation, which owned Cartier's, Valentino's and Mark Cross stores.

STANLEY, JOHN AND SANDRA. The Stanleys owned their first Rhodesian Ridgeback in 1977. He became a multiple Group-winning, nationally ranked specimen in the United States and Canada and a Register of Merit Producer.

Their Mshindaji Kennels has produced more than 125 champions in the United States, and Sandra has been Breeder of the Year 1992, 1994 and 1995, and several times in the 1980s. Their dogs have served as foundation stock for many successful kennels today.

John and Sandra Stanley reside in Middleboro, Massachusetts.

STANSELL, ROBIN. Robin Stansell is a breeder-exhibitor of French Bulldogs. Her kennel name, the Royal Regiment, was founded on a dog acquired from Suzi and Abe Segal, Ch. Tarustrail T.N.T. The Bulldog was her original breed.

Stansell was the 1996 show chairman and is a member of the French Bulldog Club of America Specialty Guidelines Committee. She judged the first French Bulldog Regional Specialty in 1994 in Orlando, Florida. She is approved to judge seven breeds in the Non-Sporting Group.

STAUDT-CARTABONA, KAREN. A Borzoi breeder since the early 1960s, Karen Staudt-Cartabona's Majenkir Kennels has produced more than 300 American Borzoi champions. Many top kennels and Borzoi in the United States and overseas have a strong Majenkir base in their bloodlines.

Staudt-Cartabona is a life member of the Borzoi Club of America, holding various board positions over the years, including that club's AKC delegate from 1977 to 1984. She was reelected in 1993 and continues in that role. She was the cofounder of the Borzoi Club of Greater New York and the all-breed Delaware Water Gap Kennel Club. She was a cofounder and board member of the International Borzoi Council.

Staudt-Cartabona's involvement with the breed extends to Russia, where she has visited breeders and collected literature on the heritage of the breed. She is an active participant in a program to bring aid to Russian breeders and their dogs with medicine, vaccines and money.

Karen Staudt-Cartabona is also a portraitist specializing in show dogs.

STEBBINS, J. MONROE, JR. "Steb" was born in New York City, raised and educated in Bayside, Queens, where dogs played a large part in his life. He became a breeder and exhibitor of Miniature Pinschers, Cocker Spaniels and West Highland White Terriers. His great love, however, was Doberman Pinschers. He showed many Dobes of his own breeding to their championships under his kennel prefix, Stebs. In 1962 he became an

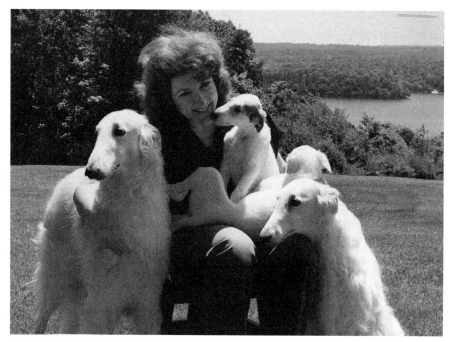

Karen Staudt-Cartabona with some of her Majenkir Borzoi.

approved professional handler and continued in that role until he joined the American Kennel Club as a field representative in 1973.

Stebbins and his wife, Natalie, had three children and several grand-children and lived in Kent, Connecticut. His kennel became the training ground for many of the top Working dog handlers in the profession today. He was known for his honesty and strong moral fiber. Stebbins died suddenly in March 1986.

STERN, ALAN J. Born in 1925 in Cambridge, Massachusetts, Alan Stern attended the Massachusetts Institute of Technology and graduated from Dartmouth in 1947. He served as an officer aboard a U.S. Navy destroyer in World War II.

From 1938 until 1976 he was a copywriter, account executive and vice-president for various advertising and public relations firms. From 1976 until 1987 he was president of The Marketing Group, Inc., a strategic marketing, public relations and advertising company. In 1987 he joined the American Kennel Club as vice-president of Communication and remained in that position until his retirement in 1991.

Stern's hobbies include animals, flying, sailing, scuba diving, photography, riding and skiing.

He has been a breeder-exhibitor of Miniature Pinschers since 1966 and acquired his first Irish Water Spaniel in 1968. It is that breed with which he is most closely associated. Although never a large-scale breeder, Alan Stern produced Group, National Specialty and many breed winners for his Whistlehill Kennel.

Stern is a member of Eastern Dog Club and Greater Venice Florida Dog Club. He is the delegate to the AKC from the Irish Water Spaniel Club of America, for which he served as president and the chairman of its Genetic Health Committee, as well as show chair and secretary. He is a member of several animal welfare groups and has written two papers on animal cruelty and on enforcing the Animal Welfare Act. He is a member of the Dog Writers' Association of America, a breed columnist for the *AKC Gazette* for twelve years and has published articles in many dog publications and in the *New York Times*.

Stern judges half the breeds in the Sporting Group and Miniature Pinschers. He lives in Sarasota, Florida, where he is on the board of Southwest Florida Judges Study Group and the Animal Health Foundation.

STEVENSON, TOM AND ANN. Tom and his late wife, Ann, were two of the most respected figures in the dog sport. Both distinguished themselves as superlative judges and are most closely identified with the Santa Barbara Kennel Club all-breed show that they ran and developed into one of the most prestigious events of its kind in America. The Stevensons began the practice of engaging foreign judges for their annual panels and built Santa Barbara into one of the largest shows, certainly the largest on the West Coast. They bred and exhibited Poodles, and Tom became a professional handler after he returned from a stint in the navy in World War II. The couple met in 1948. Tom began judging in 1964 and is now a judge emeritus. Ann started her judging assignments in 1965 and continued until her death several years ago.

STIFEL, WILLIAM F. William Frederick Stifel, fourteenth president of the American Kennel Club, joined the AKC staff in 1957. He became executive secretary in 1964, executive vice-president in 1976 and president in 1978, retiring in 1987. He served on the AKC's board of directors from 1977 until 1990.

Born in Toledo, Ohio, Stifel studied at Western Reserve Academy and Harvard University. He married Carolyn Graham of New Orleans in 1957. They have two daughters.

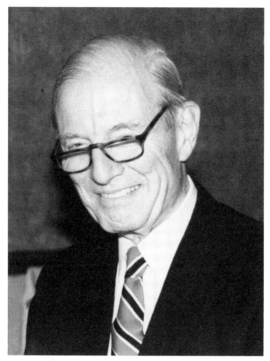

William F. Stifel, former president of the American
Kennel Club.

Bill Stifel was chairman of the Beagle Advisory Committee from 1969 until 1977. He represented the AKC at the first World Conference of Kennel Clubs in London in 1978 and at the Second World Conference in Edinburgh in 1981. He was chairman of the third World Conference, hosted by the AKC in Philadelphia in 1984.

He was delegate of the San Francisco Dog Training Club from 1970 until 1971 and of the Greater St. Louis Training Club from 1977 until 1987. He has been a member of Westminster Kennel Club since 1976 and of Westchester Kennel Club since 1980. He was founding president of the American Kennel Club Foundation that in 1980 established the Dog Museum.

Bill and Carolyn Stifel live in Irvington-on-Hudson, New York.

STOECKER, HENRY. Born in 1903 in Germany, Henry Stoecker had a very successful career as a professional handler, being especially well known for his ability with Poodles. After his retirement from handling, Stoecker

179

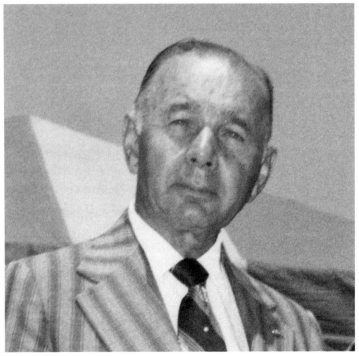

Henry H. Stoecker, all-breed judge and former professional handler.

developed a reputation as one of the sport's legendary judges. During his years as a handler, he operated from a base in Holmdel, New Jersey, where his Stoeckersburg Kennel was known for producing Boxers and Doberman Pinschers. His first judging assignment was in 1934, but he began judging in earnest after his service in the U.S. Army where, naturally, he trained dogs.

He became an all-rounder and was much in demand throughout America and around the world. His judging credits include many of the most prestigious assignments anywhere. He had the coveted honor of judging Best in Show at Westminster in 1979. He is now retired.

STREICHER, JUDSON L. Known for his Galandjud Boxers, Jud Streicher spends the workweeks on Wall Street and his weekends either fishing, golfing or involved with either Westchester Kennel Club or Westminster Kennel Club. He serves on the boards of both clubs and is the delegate to the AKC from Westchester. He has been involved in Obedience for many years and judges all Obedience classes.

STROH, BETTY. One of the early advocates of German Wirehaired Pointers in the United States, Betty Stroh's Hilltop Kennels were the foundation of many important kennels for the breed. She bred Ch. Hilltop's SS Cheesecake, CD, owned by Patricia Laurans, the top winning German Wirehaired Pointer bitch in the history of the breed up to the 1970s.

SUNDSTROM, HAROLD W. Hal Sundstrom is an award-winning purebred dog writer, author, international editorial consultant and host-director of dog fancier video productions. His byline has been familiar throughout the dog Fancy, and he edited and published breed and all-breed publications in Hawaii, Arizona and Virginia. In 1993 he received the Dog Writers' Association of America's Distinguished Service Award. He is a past DWAA president and currently serves as vice-chairman of the Dog Writers' Educational Trust.

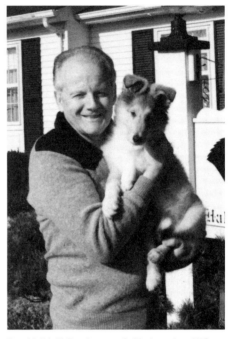

Harold "Hal" Sundstrom, Collie breeder, AKC delegate and past president of Dog Writers' Association of America.

Sundstrom has bred and exhibited Halamar Collies since 1970. He is an experienced match and sweepstakes judge, officer and director of Specialty and all-breed clubs and state councils of dog clubs, show and symposium chair. He is a past president and director of the Collie Club of America and its nonprofit breed research foundation. He is a delegate to the AKC from that club as well.

During his career Sundstrom was Foreign Service information officer with the United States Embassies in Tokyo, Jakarta and Seoul. He was vice-president of the Eisenhower People to People Program in Kansas City and Copenhagen. He was a speech writer and public affairs consultant to the commander in chief of the U.S. Pacific Forces, assistant secretary of the United States International Trade Commission and vice-president of the Export-Import Bank of the United States. Currently he is president of Halamar Publications, International Editorial Consultants in Easley, South Carolina.

In addition to his love of dogs Hal Sundstrom's interests include touring and hiking in national and regional parks and monuments; conservation and preservation of historic properties (landscapes and buildings); domestic and foreign travel; still and video photography of landscapes, people and places; literature; music; college and professional baseball and football; horse racing and the Indy 500. He is a member of Colonial Williamsburg, the Civil War Trust and South Carolina Historic Society.

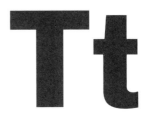

TACKER, JOSEPH C. A retired commercial airline pilot, Joe Tacker is one of the small number of AKC-approved all-breed judges. He began his involvement with dogs in 1951 with a Cocker Spaniel bitch, who never won a point. The next year he bought a show-quality animal that started him toward show ring success. Tacker lived in Hawaii for many years and realized that a coated breed was not easy to maintain, so he became active in Boxers in 1958.

Joe Tacker also owned English Setters and Norwich Terriers after a move to the mainland. He now lives in Monterey, California.

TARRANT, BILL. In 1981 Bill Tarrant became the first person named Writer of the Year by the Dog Writers' Association of America. He repeated this honor in 1983. Subsequently that award was discontinued. He is the only person asked by a British monarch to write a story about the royal kennels (1975). He was also named Writer of the Year by the Outdoor Writers' Association of America in 1980, the only dog writer to be selected.

Tarrant has been a columnist since 1973, writing in *Field & Stream* magazine and is the author of eleven books. He was nominated for a Pulitzer prize in 1996 for his family dog book, *The Magic of Dogs* (New York: Lyons & Burford, 1995). He is a nationally acknowledged crusader for humane gun dog training.

Bill Tarrant resides in Las Vegas, Nevada.

TAUSKEY, RUDOLPH WILLIAM. A unique artist and one of the greatest photographers of dogs the United States has ever known, Rudolph Tauskey was the undisputed master of his day. He was the only official photographer ever retained by the American Kennel Club, a position he held from 1924 to 1942.

Tauskey was born in Budapest, Hungary, in 1888. At age seventeen he emigrated to the United States and was introduced to photography while serving in the United States Army during World War I.

Following the war Tauskey worked with photographers in New York and at the same time became involved with dogs. He raised German Shepherd Dogs and English Springer Spaniels under the prefix Ruann. In 1916 he married Anna Peters and the family lived in Saddle River, New Jersey,

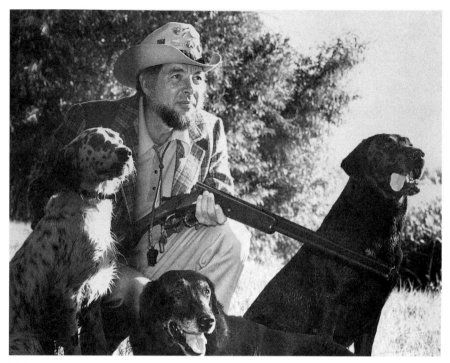

Bill Tarrant, outdoor writer, author of eleven books, with three of his hunting companions.

for forty-six years. At his spacious home and grounds landscaped with beautiful trees he photographed the famous dogs of the era.

After his death in 1979 the photographs and negatives were donated by his family to the AKC Library. Some of the pictures are only identified by their breeds. Others give the names of the dogs and owners. Tauskey developed his own film and was an expert retoucher. He was not averse to presenting the owners with photos of their dogs in their best light, but as a record of four decades his vast collection cannot be equaled.

TAYLOR, R. WILLIAM. Born in Winnipeg, Canada, Bill Taylor's interest in purebred dogs started as a child. He owned his first Pekingese in 1943, exhibited his first dog in 1944 and bred his first litter of Pekingese in 1945. Fifty years later he is still at the top of the Pekingese breed and he has won the Pedigree award for top Canadian breeder of champions in 1992 and 1993.

Taylor made his debut as a judge in Canada in 1954. Starting in 1967 he lived in England for seven years, where he exhibited and continued his judging career. In partnership with Nigel Aubrey-Jones they had one of the leading kennels in the United Kingdom, owning in one year the top winning Pekingese as well as the foremost Pekingese kennel. During the years he lived in England he was approved to judge on the championship show level in thirty breeds.

In the seventies Taylor returned to Canada and became an all-breed judge there and has officiated at many important shows worldwide. He is a popular judge in the United States and Great Britain. He has judged Best in Show at the Melbourne Royal in Australia and the Milan International show in Italy. He has judged the Toy Group both at Crufts and at Westminster, perhaps the first time that one person has held the honor of fulfilling both assignments.

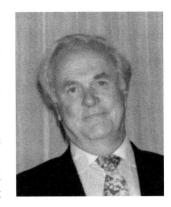

R. William Taylor, noted judge and partner with Nigel Aubrey-Jones in the St. Aubrey-Elsdon Kennel of top winning Pekingese.

In both the United States and Canada the St. Aubrey-Elsdon Kennel has created and broken more records than any other Pekingese kennel. The partnership imported and later sold the top winning Pekingese of all time, Am., Can. Ch. Chik T'Sun of Caversham who was Best in Show at Westminster in 1960. It also bred another Westminster winner, Am., Can. Ch. St. Aubrey Dragonora of Elsdon who took the top award in 1982. In all, Mr. Taylor has bred or cobred close to 150 champions in that breed.

Taylor has also been successfully involved with all varieties of Poodles, Brussels Griffons, Shih Tzus, Yorkshire Terriers, Pomeranians, Smooth Fox Terriers and Pembroke Welsh Corgis. Also in partnership with Nigel Aubrey-Jones he imported two Best in Show winning Welsh Terriers.

THOMSON, PETER. Seventy-two years ago Peter Thomson won his first Best in Show with "Nollie," a Smooth Fox Terrier he was given as a fifth birthday present. Since then he has owned, bred and won with many breeds, including Smooth Fox Terriers, Standard Smooth Dachshunds, Australian Terriers, Scottish Terriers, Whippets, Australian Cattle Dogs, Pekingese, Pugs, and for the last thirty-five years Pembroke Welsh Corgis in conjunction with his wife, Helen. Helen is a Cardigan and Pembroke Welsh Corgi judge.

Although his main love is dogs, Thomson has had many other sporting and breeding interests over the years. These include surf lifesaving and amateur swimming coach. In Australia surf lifesavers are an elite corps of volunteers. He raised poultry, pigeons and cage birds. He showed, bred and judged stud cattle. He currently has a stud of Border Leicester Sheep and breeds Magpie Pigeons.

Thomson served in the armed services for six years during World War II, where he was a POW in Germany for four of those years. Upon his return to Australia he became involved with two of the canine publications there. He was appointed to the committee of the Kennel Control Council and served in that capacity until 1962. In 1970 he was transferred by his business, an international transport company, to California, where he became chief executive officer. He retired as an executive in 1983 and returned to Australia but continued on the board of the parent company until his retirement in 1988 on his seventieth birthday.

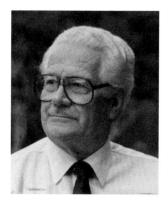

Peter Thomson, judge of all breeds in the United States; resident of Australia.

Peter Thomson has been an all-breed judge in Australia since 1952 and attained AKC approval for all breeds in 1979. While living in California he was delegate to the AKC from Golden Gate Kennel Club.

He has judged at many of the world's most prestigious shows, including the Sydney Royal, Melbourne Royal and Brisbane Royal. He has judged at most of the major shows in the United States, including three times at Westminster, and he has judged extensively in many other parts of the world.

THORNTON, KIM CAMPBELL. Kim Thornton, who was editor of *Dog Fancy* magazine from 1988 until 1996 when she left to freelance, grew up with dogs that included an Old English Sheepdog, two German Shepherd Dogs and several mixed breeds at various times.

After earning a bachelor's degree in journalism from the University of Oklahoma in 1982, Thorton and her husband moved to California, where she was hired as an editorial assistant at *Dog Fancy*. She now writes full-time, primarily about pets. Her current dog is an eleven-year-old retired racing Greyhound named Savanna.

In addition to dogs, Kim Thorton enjoys cats, reading, traveling and scuba diving. She and her husband live in Lake Forest, California.

THRELFALL, MARK E. Mark Threlfall began his career in dogs in 1968 and finished his first champion when he was seventeen years old. Having chosen to become a professional handler, he apprenticed to William Trainor and to Bob and Jane Forsyth.

In 1975 he married Bonnie Proctor, who came from a family of professional handlers and dog breeders. Her father, Harry Proctor, was well known for showing English Cockers and other Sporting dogs. Her late brother, Scott, was a professional handler, as is her sister, Patricia Proctor Jenner. The Threlfalls have one son, Evan Michael, born in 1982.

Mark was the youngest board member and subsequently the youngest president of the Professional Handlers' Association. He has won Bests in Show with dogs from all seven Variety Groups. He exhibited the Top Dog all-breeds in 1992 to a record of 76 Bests in Show and 123 Group firsts. That dog, an English Springer Spaniel, Ch. Salilyn's Condor, won Best in Show at Westminster in 1993 with Threlfall handling. He won the Gaines FIDO award for Handler of the Year in 1992, and he has twice been the handler of the Quaker Oats awards winner.

He has bred Smooth Fox Terriers and English Cocker Spaniels with Bonnie at their Edgewood Farm Kennel in Pennsylvania.

In 1995 he retired from professional handling and is employed by the AKC as director of Customer Services in Durham, North Carolina.

TIETJEN, SARI BREWSTER. Sari Tietjen was born into a dog show family. Her mother, Mary Brewster, bred many breeds of dogs at her Robwood Kennels. Her sister, Joy Brewster, is an all-breed professional handler. Tietjen showed her first dog when she was five years old and at age seven had her first breeder-owner-handled champion. She specializes in Japanese Chin but became familiar with Cocker Spaniels, English Springer Spaniels, Shetland Sheepdogs, Collies, Great Pyrenees, Borzois, Beagles, Dachshunds, Pekingese, Pomeranians, Pugs, Italian Greyhounds, Poodles and Dalmatians through her mother's influence.

During the time Sari Tietjen showed dogs she was the breeder-owner-handler of Group placing Chins for five straight generations. She still owns Japanese Chins, occasionally breeding and showing to maintain her line.

She has been an approved AKC judge for more than twenty-five years. Presently she judges all Hound, Toy and Non-Sporting breeds. She has judged throughout the United States, as well as in Canada, England, Denmark, Finland, Russia, Venezuela, Brazil and Puerto Rico.

Tietjen is a professional writer. Her articles and interviews have appeared in many canine publications. She has been a weekly columnist for *Dog News* since 1988 and formerly wrote a weekly column for her local newspaper entitled "Canine Corner."

She is the author of five published books and is presently writing a book about the Japanese Chin.

Sari Tietjen has won Gaines FIDO awards for Dog Writer of the Year and Dog Woman of the Year. She also won *Kennel Review*'s WINKIE for Outstanding Journalist, and she has won various awards from the Dog Writers' Association of America.

TINGLEY, ARTHUR AND MARY LOU. Art and Mary Lou Tingley began their association with Briards in 1957 with the purchase of a pet for their daughter. With no intention of showing they took their pet to Obedience classes and in four trials completed her CD at the age of fifteen months. They became so fascinated by the breed that they bought a young male from France and an American-bred bitch. These two became the foundation stock for Briards Chez Phydeau. In 1978 Art showed a bitch, Ch. Jennie del Pastre, to Best in Show, the first time a Briard bitch has ever taken a top award in the United States.

A moderate breeding program, twenty-two litters over the next thirty-eight years, brought them more than fifty champions, including several who went on to win Group and Best in Show awards. Art Tingley has served as president and director of Sussex Hills Kennel Club, president and show chairman for Schooley's Mountain Kennel Club, director and AKC delegate for the Briard Club of America and director and eye clinic chairman for the Atlantic States Briard Club.

Mary Lou has served as director, secretary and president of the Briard Club of America, president of the Atlantic States Briard Club, show chairman for the Sussex Hills Kennel Club and show secretary and president of Schooley's Mountain Kennel Club. She began judging in 1968 and retired in 1991. Her varied assignments included several in Europe and two Briard Club of America National Specialties.

Their Chez Phydeau Briards can be found in the pedigrees of many of the major kennels in the breed today.

TIPTON, E. W. "Tip" Tipton was an all-round judge and breeder of English Setters and Pointers, but it was as a breeder-exhibitor of Miniature Pinschers that he was best known. His Rebel Roc kennels produced many top winners, but the most famous was his Ch. Rebel Roc's Casanova von Kurt. His call name was "Little Daddy," named after one of the characters in the play *Cat on a Hot Tin Roof* (with poetic license), according to Tip, who showed him throughout his remarkable career. He retired the dog with his seventy-fifth Best in Show in 1962.

Tipton was a lifelong resident of Kingsport, Tennessee. He served in World War II and following his discharge entered the insurance business from which he retired in 1977.

He first started judging in 1957 and became an all-rounder in 1982.

He was renowned in dog show circles for his humor and his ability to make exhibitors feel at ease. One could always count on Tip for a good joke, either in the ring or outside. He was respected for his opinion, and he was always in great demand as a judge. He died in 1987.

TOMITA, RICHARD. Rick Tomita came into Shiba Inus having already been successful in Boxers. He produced more than 100 champions in that breed. He imported fifteen Shibas from several kennels so that he could keep the gene pool broad. One of his top imports, Ch. Katsuranishike of Oikawa House, ROM, finished his championship title the first year that Shibas were recognized by AKC. Remarkably, he was eight years old.

Rick is no longer involved with Shibas, but his imports continue to appear in the pedigrees of some of the country's top winning dogs. Rick is the co-owner of J & B Pet Supply Company.

TRAINOR, ELIZABETH F., VMD. Betty Fortune earned her veterinary degree at the University of Pennsylvania, when the number of women veterinarians was very limited. There she had been elected to the honorary veterinary fraternity of Phi Zeta in her third year and was awarded the Borden Award and the Leonard Pearson Prize at graduation. She served an internship and residency at Angell Memorial Animal Hospital in Boston, Massachusetts, after which she joined the regular staff there. While at Angell, she pioneered in veterinary nursing, establishing a formal nurses training program, and wrote their first *Manual of Veterinary Nursing*. She served on the staff for eight years.

Dr. Trainor showed her first Doberman Pinscher in conformation as well as in Obedience in the early 1950s. She became seriously interested in purebred dogs after her marriage in 1957 to professional handler Bill Trainor. She spent some time away from veterinary practice attending shows regularly and developing an insight into breeders' and exhibitors' problems. Having developed a whole new concept of the application of veterinary medicine to problems peculiar to those engaged in breeding and showing dogs, she then went into private practice and for many years dealt primarily with breeder and exhibitor clientele. She later limited her practice to canine reproduction. A member of the Society for Theriogenology, she established an AKC-approved canine frozen semen facility in Oxford, Massachusetts, under license to Canine Cryobank of California.

For a number of years, Dr. Trainor was actively engaged lecturing at breeder seminars throughout the country on the subject of canine structure as well as on canine reproduction and the use of cooled and frozen semen. She has been the recipient of the Gaines FIDO for Woman of the Year.

In December 1997 Bill and Betty will have been married for forty years. They have two grown children, Shawn and Sharon, and three grand-children.

TRAINOR, WILLIAM J. Bill Trainor began his career in dogs in 1946, breeding Great Danes. He had the eighth Great Dane in the United States to win a Utility degree. He began in Obedience, where he met his future wife, veterinarian Elizabeth A. Fortune.

In 1950 Bill was licensed as an all-breed professional handler by the AKC, and for the next 44 years he attended more than 100 shows per year, handling an average of from 10 to 30 dogs at a show. He was president of the Professional Handlers Association for eleven years. During his career he won hundreds of Bests in Show with dogs from all seven Variety Groups, including two Westminster top awards, first in 1979 with the Irish Water Spaniel, Ch. Oaktree's Irishtocrat and then in 1982 with the Pekingese, Ch. St. Aubrey Dragonora of Elsdon. Both dogs were owned by Mrs. Anne Snelling. He retired as a handler in 1994, after taking a Best in Show with a Portuguese Water Dog that he and his wife had bred and raised, owned by Joan Hawkins.

Trainor was honored by Gaines with FIDO's Dogdom's Man of the Year and Handler of the Year award twice. He received awards from *Kennel Review* as the person making "outstanding contributions" to the sport of dogs. While he was president of PHA, that organization was awarded special recognition for making "outstanding contributions" in the sport. In 1994 he was inducted into the Ken-L Ration Hall of Fame.

He began judging in 1995 and at present is licensed for twenty-five breeds in all seven Groups.

In addition to handling, he and Betty have bred more than twenty-five litters of Poodles in all three varieties, as well as Beagles, German Short-haired Pointers and currently Portuguese Water Dogs.

His hobbies are landscaping and gardening. More than twenty gardens surround his home, including a fifty-bush rose garden and extensive iris and lily plantings, perennials and a small vegetable garden.

TREEN, ALFRED AND ESMERALDA. Al and Esme Treen are familiar faces in dog show circles far and wide. They are longtime breeders of Dalmatians, with their most famous dog being Ch. Coachman's Chuck-A-Luck,

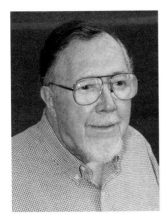

Alfred E. Treen, former AKC board member, Dalmatian fancier, judge and chairman of the Dog Writers' Educational Trust.

who contributed strongly to many breed lines. They have written many articles for dog magazines and newspapers and are coauthors of two books, *The Dalmatian, Coach Dog, Firehouse Dog* (New York: Howell Book House, 1980) and *The New Dalmatian* (New York: Howell Book House, 1992). Al has served on the Dalmatian Club of America's board of directors, as president and as the club's AKC delegate. He is presently the delegate from Waukesha Kennel Club. Both Treens are active in that all-breed club, bringing their annual show to national recognition. Both Al and Esme are members of the Dog Writers' Association of America from which they have won six awards for excellence in writing. Al is also chairman of the board of the Dog Writers' Educational Trust, which is dedicated to helping worthy students with college scholarships.

Al started judging in 1965 and is an AKC-approved judge of all Hounds, Terriers, Toys and Non-Sporting dogs. Esme began in 1969 and is approved to judge all Sporting and Non-Sporting breeds, and half the Toy breeds. She also judges all Obedience classes.

They both have judged the National Specialty for the Dalmatian Club of America several times and have judged nationals for several other breeds. Their judging has taken them to a dozen different countries on six continents.

Esme grew up in a house in which dogs always played a part. Her mother bred Toy Boston Terriers, a classification now discontinued. She had dogs all her life except during the time she was in college and working at her career as Midwestern editor of *Mademoiselle* magazine.

Al got his first dog after he and Esme were married. It was a Cocker Spaniel, the most popular breed in America at that time. That did not last long, since the dog attacked their son. After one more trial with a Boxer, they decided that Dalmatians would be their breed.

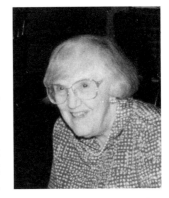

Esme Treen, writer, judge and founder of Waukesha Kennel Club.

At the time they were living in Houston, Texas, where they joined the Houston Kennel Club. They offered conformation lessons for the club, and Esme began her interest in becoming an Obedience instructor and later judge.

Following a transfer to southern Illinois the couple returned to their original home in Milwaukee, where they have remained ever since. They were the founders of the Waukesha Kennel Club. Al was elected president and has remained in that position for thirty years. The club became a member club of the AKC in 1968, and he has been its only delegate. He served on the AKC's board of directors for seven years, from 1978 until 1985. Esme served as delegate from the Idaho Capital City Kennel Club from 1983 until 1993.

Esme was instrumental in the formation of two Obedience clubs in the Milwaukee area, and in 1984 she received the D'Ambrisi award in Obedience, an honor she cherishes because it is determined by a vote of one's peers.

In the early 1960s Esme assisted the late Azalea Gascoigne Doggett in bringing the Bichon Frise to this country. She helped organize the Bichon Frise Club of America, wrote the original Standard for the breed and served on the club's board of directors for the first two years of its existence.

She was instrumental in forming the Humane Animal Welfare Society in Waukesha, and she served on its board of directors for about five years. Al served on its board for three years.

Both Al and Esme have been recognized by the AKC for twenty-five years of continuous service, he as a delegate and judge, she as a judge and show chairman.

TROTTER, CHARLES E. "Chuck" Trotter is president of the Mid-South Aluminum Company in Nashville, Tennessee. About the same time as he began his employment in the late 1950s he started showing and breeding Afghan Hounds under the Silverstone prefix. He also raised German Shepherd Dogs and his enjoyment of the sport led him to become an all-breed professional handler. He turned to judging in 1980 and is currently approved by the AKC for all Hound, Working, Non-Sporting and Herding breeds. In 1997 he judged the Working Group at Westminster.

He has been a member of the Nashville Kennel Club for thirty-seven years and served as its president for five years among other offices during his thirty years on the board.

Trotter's other interests include fishing and hunting as well as boating and tour biking on his Harley motorcycle. He enjoys cooking down-home

Southern food for his new bride, Pat Craige Trotter, whom he married in 1994. Trotter has a son and daughter and two grandchildren.

The couple enjoy the theater and are supporters of the Tennessee Performing Arts Center.

TROTTER, PATRICIA CRAIGE. Pat showed her first dog, a Cocker Spaniel, in 1947 as a child living in Norfolk, Virginia. Within a few years she had dedicated her life to improving her favorite breed—the Norwegian Elkhound—a love affair that still continues. Trotter has a bachelor of science degree from William and Mary College in Norfolk and a master of arts degree from the Monterey Institute of International Studies. She was a history teacher in California for more than thirty years at the same time that she was breeding, conditioning and showing her dogs. She was also president of Del Monte Kennel Club for three years.

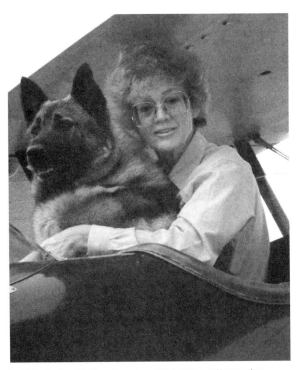

Patricia Craige Trotter, breeder of top winning Norwegian Elkhounds, lecturer, judge and author with Ch. Vin-Melca's Bombardier.

For almost thirty years her Vin-Melca Norwegian Elkhounds exerted a significant impact on the American show scene, so it comes as no surprise that their most significant permanent contribution was to the breed's gene pool. Ch. Vin-Melca's Vagabond was number one dog, all breeds in 1970 and two of his grandchildren ranked number two all breeds. They were the top winning male in the breed, Ch. Vin-Melca's Nimbus and the top bitch, Ch. Vin-Melca's Calista. Ch. Vin-Melca's Howdy Rowdy is the number one Hound sire with 166 champion progeny and Ch. Vin-Melca's Last Call is the top brood bitch with 27 champion offspring.

Pat Trotter garnered ten Group I firsts placements at Westminster and a number of Quaker Oats victories. Her last Quaker Oats winner was Ch. Vin-Melca's Bombadier in 1992. He was the sire of two-time Westminster Group winner and the 1993 Quaker Oats winner, Ch. Vin-Melca's Marketta. Trotter became a member of the Quaker Oats Hall of Fame in 1990 and was Gaines Dog Woman of the Year in 1991. She is also the recipient of awards from *Kennel Review* as breeder-owner-handler and was elected to the Hall of Fame.

She began judging the Hound breeds in 1993 and is the author of *Born to Win* (Wilsonville, Oregon: Doral Publishing, Inc., 1996). After her marriage to Chuck Trotter in 1994 she moved to Nashville, Tennessee.

Vv-Ww

VAN ALLEN, BONNIE FISCHER. Bonnie Van Allen owned the first Australian Cattle dog to attain her AKC championship in the fall of 1980. Fischer and her son, Todd, owned some of the top winning Aussies, starting in the late 1970s. Their brood bitch, Fischer Jarmo Blue Anna, CD, is in the background of many of the foundation Australian Cattle Dogs in the United States.

VESLEY, ROBERTA. A native of Long Island, Roberta Vesley has been a breeder and exhibitor of Soft Coated Wheaten Terriers from 1969, prior to the breed's official AKC recognition in 1973. She is the author of *The Complete Soft Coated Wheaten Terrier* (New York: Howell Book House, 1991).

Vesley joined the staff of the American Kennel Club in 1975 and served as its library director from 1980 until 1991. She was a founding member and past president of the Soft Coated Wheaten Terrier Club of Metropolitan New York, a director of the Soft Coated Wheaten Terrier Club of America and a director and secretary of Long Island Kennel Club. She has been a guest curator for the Dog Museum and has written on dogs for *World Book, Readers Digest* and the *AKC Gazette.* Vesley is a member of the Dog Writers' Association of America.

Roberta Vesley and husband, Alan, have two daughters and live in Port Washington, New York.

VOGELS, CINDY. Together with her mother, Jackie Gottlieb, Cindy Vogels has shown Soft Coated Wheaten Terriers since 1968. Under the Andover prefix they have bred more than 100 American champions, including multiple Specialty, Group and Best in Show winners. They have had many top producers, including the top producing Terrier dam of all time.

Vogels has also bred champion Kerry Blue, Welsh and Norfolk Terriers.

She is past president of the Soft Coated Wheaten Terrier Club of America and was a founding member of the SCWTC of Metropolitan New York and Greater Denver. She is a member of the Providence County and Cen-Tex Kennel Clubs. She is a lifetime member of Flatirons Kennel Club and serves on its show committee. She is also a board member and show chairman of the Evergreen County Kennel Club, Colorado.

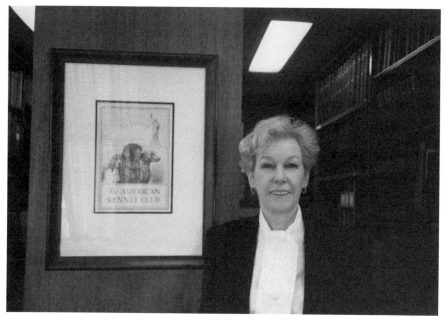

Roberta Vesley, former AKC librarian, author and Soft Coated Wheaten Terrier fancier.

She is an approved judge of several of the Terrier breeds.

Married for nearly twenty years, Vogel and her husband, David, have one son. They also raise and show Morgan horses, also under the Andover prefix. They reside in Littleton, Colorado.

WAGNER, MAZIE. Mrs. John (Mazie) Wagner, owner with her husband, John, of the famous Mazelaine Kennels, bred top winning and producing Boxers for thirty years, starting in the 1930s. They bred more than 100 champions, among them some of the all-time greats in the breed, including the 1947 Westminster Best in Show Winner.

Mrs. Wagner was a judge for many years, her last assignment being in 1969. She was also active in the American Boxer Club and was the founder of the Mid-West Boxer Club in 1936.

WALKER, HELENE WHITEHOUSE. Mrs. Walker founded the sport of Obedience in America in 1933 with the first all-breed Obedience test that she organized at her father's estate in Mt. Kisco, New York. In 1935 she wrote a booklet called *Obedience Tests: Procedure for Judge, Handler, and Show Giving Club*. The booklet was submitted to the AKC and became the forerunner to the present official Obedience regulations.

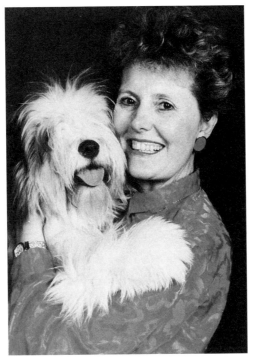

Chris Walkowicz, award-winning author, columnist
and breeder of Bearded Collies.

After AKC recognition of Obedience as a regular event, in 1936 Mrs. Walker made her famous ten-week "Trailer Trek" from Ohio to California with Miss Blanche Saunders and three Standard Poodles. The pair toured shows, dog clubs, towns and villages to introduce Obedience to the public.

In 1983 Mrs. Walker was honored with a Gaines FIDO award for outstanding service and contributions to the advancement of Obedience training and competition.

Mrs. Walker died in 1986 at age eighty-six.

WALKOWICZ, CHRIS. Chris Walkowicz and her husband, Ed, began showing German Shepherd Dogs in 1965. She discovered Bearded Collies in 1977, and they have been breeding and showing Beardies ever since. With limited breeding they have produced thirty-five champions, seven Register of Merit producers, one Obedience Trial champion and Beardies that have achieved nineteen Obedience titles and twenty-three Herding titles.

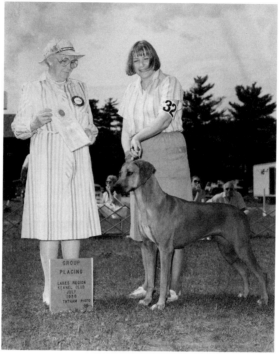

Margaret "Peg" Walton, veteran Basset Hound breeder and judge of all Hounds, awarding a Group third to the Rhodesian Ridgeback, Ch. Mshindaji Special K, owned, bred and shown by Sandra Stanley, whose biography appears in an earlier chapter.

Walkowicz has served as Bearded Collie Club of America recording secretary and has been on the board of directors. She has written the Bearded Collie breed column in the *AKC Gazette* and frequently contributes to that magazine. She has received the BCCA Ian Morrison Outstanding Member award and the Chicagoland BCC Lifetime Achievement Award. She and her husband are active in several local dog clubs and she is vice-president of Annual Affairs for the National War Dog Memorial Project.

Ed Walkowicz was a professional handler, retiring in 1985, and he now devotes his time to the dogs and dog shows at which he often stewards.

As a professional writer and author, Chris Walkowicz has written or coauthored seven books on dogs, many of which have received national recognition. She has also been awarded the Dog Writers' Association of America Distinguished Service Award and has received the Quad-City Times

Alice French Award for Quad-City authors. She has written more than 700 articles and columns in all the major canine publications.

In 1995 Chris Walkowicz was approved to judge Bearded Collies, German Shepherd Dogs and Shetland Sheepdogs. She was also the recipient of the 1996 Gaines FIDO for Dog Woman of the Year.

WALTON, MARGARET "PEG." One of the best-known Basset Hound breeders in the United States from the 1940s through the 1970s was Peg Walton. Her Lyn-Mar Acres Kennel bred more than seventy-five champions. Walton grew up with horses and dogs. Her grandfather bred coach and hackney horses. Her father raised standardbreds and had a herd of registered Jersey cattle. Her husband came into the marriage with a pack of Beagles and Peg presented him with a Basset Hound as a surprise in 1943.

Peg Walton was show chairman of Trenton Kennel Club for nine years during the period in which that club's annual show was expanding to one of the largest in the East. Her last stint in that role was in 1971. She is an approved judge of all Hounds, Working and Non-Sporting breeds and Toy Poodles. She lives in Easthampton, New Jersey.

WARD, JOHN S. Jack Ward was chairman of the board of the American Kennel Club from 1992 until 1994. He was first elected to the board of directors in 1974 and had been treasurer of the organization since 1979. He is a delegate to AKC from Mt. Vernon Dog Training Club.

Ward and his late wife, Norma, bred and showed Cocker Spaniels in conformation and Obedience for forty years. He has been an Obedience judge since 1962 and has served as a member of every AKC advisory committee since 1966.

Ward received a bachelor of science degree in chemical engineering from the University of Notre Dame. He served in the U.S. Navy during World War II, worked as a research chemist and as a communications engineer in private industry after the war. Before his retirement he was employed by the federal government in Washington, D.C. He lives in Great Falls, Virginia.

Jack Ward is a member of American Spaniel Club, and past president of the Association of Obedience Clubs and Judges.

WARD, ROBERT AND DOLLY. Bob and Dolly Ward met at UCLA. Their extracurricular activities while at college included wrestling, various sports, and their societal lives. The couple married in 1942 just before Lieutenant Ward went overseas. Eventually they moved their young family of two

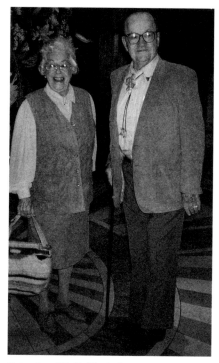

Robert and Dolly Ward, Samoyed breeders,
judges and authors of three revisions of *The
Complete Samoyed.*

daughters to a rural setting in the San Fernando Valley known as Hidden
Hills, where they could raise Morgan horses and dogs.

After several litters of Samoyeds, exhibiting to championships, running
sled teams, spinning dog hair, adding Poodles and Pembroke Welsh Corgis
to their dog experiences, they were deeply involved in the dog game.

Both were presidents of all-breed kennel clubs and of the Samoyed
Club of America. Later they became AKC judges until Dolly had been
approved for four Groups and Bob had five. They found their hobby of
dogs for the family had become a profession. This sent them around the
world by invitation, judging their favorite creatures while their children
married and began anew.

Lindy raised their grandchildren and Mardee continued with the
Samoyeds under the prefix Hoof N' Paw. Mardee Ward-Fanning also became an AKC judge. She campaigned their Ch. Hoof N' Paw's A Rose Is A

Rose with Robert Chaffin handling for Jeffrey and Nan Eisley Bennett to number one Samoyed and one of the top twenty Working Dogs in 1996.

The Wards have done three revisions on their book *The Complete Samoyed* (New York: Howell Book House, 1997).

WATSON, CRAIG. Craig resides on a small farm on Harstine Island in the State of Washington. He has been involved with dogs his entire life, owning purebred Australian Cattle Dogs for nine years and AKC-registered Aussies for six. He actively competes in all the Herding Trials held by various organizations, including the AKC. His dog, Solo's Blue Banjo, was the first Australian Cattle Dog to earn an ASCA Working Trial championship. Winner of thirty-one Highs in Trial and holder of more Herding titles than any other Australian Cattle Dog in history, Banjo was the top winning working Australian Cattle Dog of 1994 and 1995.

Watson uses his dogs to manage a flock of Barbado, Blackbelly, Dorset and Cheviot sheep. The dogs help in rotating pasture, gathering, sorting, leading, trimming, drenching, vaccinating and lambing.

He is currently vice-president of the Australian Cattle Dog Club of America, president of the All-Breed Herding Club of Western Washington, vice-president of the Cascade Australian Cattle Dog Club, chairman of the AKC National Herding Championship Committee, site director for AKC Herding judge seminars and a member of the national club's herding committee.

WAY, SHAROL CANDACE "CANDY". Candy Way, a native of San Diego, California, and a history and geology graduate of San Diego State University got into dogs in 1968 with Saint Bernards and then Great Pyrenees. Looking for something smaller, she got her first Soft Coated Wheaten Terrier in 1978. Her foundation bitch, Am., Bah. Ch. Gleanngay Holly Berry produced all-breed Best in Show winner Ch. Bantry Bay Gleanngay Kashmir, ROM, National Specialty Best of Breed winner Ch. Bantry Bay Kairo, ROM and numerous Specialty and top ten Terrier winners.

Way is approved to judge Wheatens and hopes to add to her roster of approved breeds over time. Professionally she is operations manager for Zeneca CRB. She is an avid world traveler, having been to Tibet, Easter Island, gorilla watching in Rwanda and other exotic places. Bird-watching, gardening and sports are her other interests. Way is also a game show fan, having made television appearances on *Tic-Tac-Dough* and *Second Chance*. She is studying for an appearance on *Jeopardy*.

Candy Way and Roger Cotton live in Cochranville, Pennsylvania, with eight Wheatens and two cats.

WEHLE, ROBERT. A legend among bird hunters and Field Trial enthusiasts, Bob Wehle has redefined the hunting Pointer to his own mold. His Elhew (Wehle spelled backward) Kennels have produced hundreds of Field Trial champions since he began breeding in 1936. He maintains kennels in western New York and in North Carolina so that he can train his dogs throughout the year.

He is a former president of Genesee Brewing Company and is an accomplished artist and sculptor in bronze. His statues of Pointers have become collectors' items. His Book, *Wing and Shot* (Hendersonville, New York: The Country Press, 1964), is considered a classic on hunting with pointing dogs. He has also produced a video about training for the field. In addition, he is an expert cook and a collector of art and antiques.

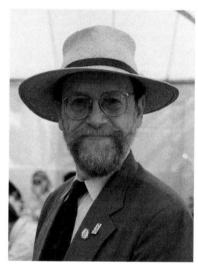

Seymour Weiss, editor, writer, judge, breeder and exhibitor of West Highland White Terriers.

WEISS, SEYMOUR. A native and lifetime resident of Brooklyn, New York, Seymour Weiss discovered the dog world as a boy and has actively participated in it for more than four decades. In that time, he has pursued a varied, fruitful career in the Fancy.

A judge of all Terrier breeds, Weiss is familiar throughout the dog Fancy for his writing. He is an executive editor with Howell Book House and has been with this highly esteemed publisher since 1971. His editorial touch is behind some of the most famous dog books in print by some of the dog Fancy's most respected authorities. He writes the West Highland White Terrier column in the *AKC Gazette* and is a feature writer for *ShowSight* magazine.

Weiss is a longtime member of the Dog Writers' Association of America and currently sits on the board of the Dog Writers' Educational Trust.

His first dogs were Kerry Blue Terriers, but they were not show dogs, so after two false starts, he gladly gave in to a weakness for the Dandie Dinmont

Terrier. His first Dandie not only became his first show dog but his first champion as well. Weiss spent more than twenty-five years with Dandies as a successful breeder-exhibitor. During this period he took up with Kerries again for a brief while and did nicely in breeding and showing.

Today in the active Fancy, Seymour Weiss is best known for West Highland White Terriers bearing his wife Helene's Glengidge prefix. He happily admits to marrying into Westies, because the couple had *her* Westies and *his* Dandies for the first fifteen years of their marriage. While Kerries and Dandies will always be special favorites, Westies have the exclusive in the couple's turn-of-the-century brownstone town house.

WELSH, DOROTHY. Dorothy Welsh was born and raised in the Chicago, Illinois area. She graduated from Northwestern University and did advanced work in guidance in Boulder, Colorado. She worked in elementary education, was a guidance counselor and had several young children's books published.

She is a second-generation dog fancier and has successfully bred a Best in Show Collie in three of the four allowable colors. Since 1969 she has concentrated on an active judging career that has taken her throughout the United States and a number of foreign countries.

Welsh has been a participating educator in numerous breed and judging seminars. She is a former state director of the Collie Club of America, a longtime officer of the Wheaton Kennel Club and has served as delegate to AKC from the Chicagoland Collie Club for more than twenty years. She is a current member of the board of directors, having been elected in 1996.

Dorothy Welsh has held all offices in the American Kennel Club Museum of the Dog. She has received a Gaines FIDO award as Woman of the Year, and in 1993 she was inducted into the Ken-L-Ration Hall of Fame.

WESTFIELD, CHARLES. A Bulldog of a man, Charlie Westfield was one of the foremost ambassadors of the breed in the 1960s and 1970s. Starting with Brookhollow Ginger, Westfield and his family, especially his daughter, Virginia, showed their Westfield Bulldogs to many Best in Show and Non-Sporting Group wins. His most famous Bulldog was Ch. Westfield Cunomorous Stone, the greatest winning Bulldog in breed history for her time. She was not only a great representative of the breed but a comical personality that endeared her to the gallery.

Charles Westfield was one of the founders of the Owner Handler Association of America, serving three terms during the 1970s as president. He lived with his family on Long Island.

WESTPHAL, PEGGY. One of America's most successful breeders of Dachshunds in all three varieties in a career that spans forty years, von Westphalen dogs are found behind many of the kennels of today, and Peggy still continues to turn out quality stock.

One of her most famous dogs, however, was not a Dachsie, but a Cocker Spaniel bitch, Ch. Sagamore Toccoa. Handled by the late Ted Young Jr., the buff Cocker won 108 Sporting Groups, including at Westminster in 1973. Other breeds with which she has been associated over the years were Airedales, Bearded Collies and Whippets. Currently, in addition to her Dachshunds she is a staunch advocate of Greyhound rescue and has several living with her.

Peggy Westphal is an excellent artist in charcoal and watercolor. Her drawings of dogs are sensitive and ethereal.

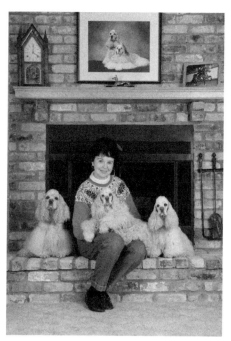

Mary Lee "Marly" Whiting, Obedience judge and instructor with her Cocker Spaniels Ch. Tainer, Ch. Bridie, UD and Tali, UD.

WHITING, MARY LEE "MARLY." Marly Whiting is an AKC Obedience judge of all classes. She has served on the AKC's Obedience Advisory Committee and has conducted training workshops throughout the United States and Canada. She served as an Obedience judge at the AKC Centennial show.

Whiting is the first recipient of a Gaines FIDO for Obedience, and she also has received the D'Ambrisi award presented by the Association of Obedience Clubs and Judges.

Her breed is the Cocker Spaniel, and she still has her original line, being the breeder of every dog she has owned except for the first one purchased as a child. She exhibits her dogs in both Obedience and conformation classes, but her primary interest is with the educated set. Her Cockers were the first two-generation breeder-handled dual champions (breed and Obedience) of any breed.

Whiting is the author of *From Cradle to College: Raising Your Puppy* and *A Utility Dog Through Class Instruction*. She has also produced a video on raising a puppy and on basic Obedience.

She conducts Canine College in Minneapolis, Minnesota, where she personally instructs nearly 300 dog owners each week in all classes from Beginners through Utility.

Another interest is in owning and exhibiting American Saddlebred horses. She has shown her horses in three-gaited and five-gaited classes.

Marly Whiting lives in Minneapolis, Minnesota.

WHITMORE, WALT AND TINA. The AfterHours Kennel of Walt and Tina Whitmore houses the current, living top American-bred, German Wire-haired Pointer sire, Ch. Shurcan Baron of AfterHours, with more than thirty-two champion get. Some of his progeny are also successful in the field.

WILKES, GARY. Gary Wilkes has worked with dogs for more than twenty years. Once the shelter manager of a small humane society, he has become a noted animal behavior specialist, award-winning author, columnist and lecturer. His primary goal is developing and teaching practical and humane training methods for pet owners.

Wilkes is the cofounder of "Clicker Training," a method that applies those goals to conditioning for dogs. He has received multiple awards from the Dog Writers Association of America and has been twice honored for his syndicated newspaper column. Wilkes also received the award for "Effective Presentation of Behavior Analysis in the Mass Media" from the Association for Behavior Analysis, an international association of experimental psychologists.

Gary Wilkes lives with his wife, Michele, in Phoenix, Arizona, along with their Australian Cattle Dog, Tug. Wilkes continues to work with animal welfare issues as a member of the board of directors of the Arizona Humane Society and is active in advancing the training and certification of Assistance and Therapy dogs.

WIMER, MRS. WILLIAM. A noted breeder and owner of Terriers, Mrs. Wimer's Poole Forge Kennel was first noted for Beagles and Harriers, although it is with Welsh, Wire and Smooth Fox Terriers, Airedales and Sealyhams that she is best remembered.

Her greatest winner was a Sealyham Terrier that Peter Green brought back from Wales, Ch. Dersade Bobby's Girl. "Binny" had a tremendous career, in the hands of Peter Green, culminating with Best in Show at Westminster in 1977.

Yy-Zz

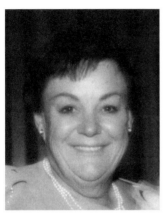

Betty Young, breeder of Cypress Woods Clumber Spaniels.

YOUNG, BETTY L. Cypress Woods Clumber Spaniels bred by Betty Young had a major influence on the Clumber in the 1970s and 1980s. She passed away in 1990, but her impact is still felt. She was a contributor in two ways: She developed a distinct line of dogs still strong and popular today, and she brought the breed to the attention of the Fancy both in and out of the ring. The dogs of her breeding were consistent winners both at all-breed shows and Specialties. She publicized these dogs, introducing them to many who had hardly ever seen a Clumber. Young was an aggressive enthusiast of the breed, extolling its praises tirelessly and stressing the Clumber Spaniel's multipurpose qualities by working her show dogs in Obedience and in the field.

Betty Young was a judge and originally bred Saint Bernards. She owned or bred five of the first seven Clumber Spaniel Best in Show dogs. Some of her best-known dogs were Ch. Cypress Woods Chesterfield, Ch. Cypress Woods Dealers Choice, Ch. Cypress Woods Chardonnay and Ch. Cypress Woods Touch of Class, UDT, JH, WDX.

ZAPHIRIS, EUGENE Z. Gene Zaphiris is the owner of Cragsmoor Kennels in Oyster Bay Cove, New York. He is the owner, breeder and handler of all breed Best in Show and National Specialty-winning Skye Terriers and Bloodhounds. He owner-handled his Skye, Ch. Finnsky Oliver to Group firsts at the 1996 Westminster Kennel Club show. He is also the owner of Best in Show and National Specialty and Westminster Best of Breed Airedale Terriers and recently English Toy Spaniels.

He was formerly advertising director of *Popular Dogs* magazine, now no longer in existence. He is the founder and editor-in-chief of the weekly newspaper, *Dog News*, and *D, The Dog News Annual*, a magazine. Zaphiris's editorial staff contains more Dog Writers' Association of America award-winning writers than any other dog publication.

He is a former trustee of the Morris Animal Foundation and currently serves on the board of St. Hubert's Giralda, Animal Shelter and Education Center.

ZIESSOW, DR. AND MRS. BERNARD. Franklin Labradors was established in 1951 by the Ziessows. The kennel has produced more than sixty-five champions, including two Field Champions, Master Hunters, a winner of nine Bests in Show and the National Specialty winner Ch. Dark Star of Franklin. They also bred and owned two-time National Specialty winner, Ch. Golden Chance of Franklin.

Mrs. Ziessow breeds the dogs, limiting herself to two or three litters a year. She is an AKC judge emerita of Sporting dogs. Dr. Ziessow is an officer and director of the Labrador Retriever Club, president of an all-breed club and is an active AKC judge of dog shows and hunting tests. He was editor of the *Official Book of the Labrador Retriever* and served as chairman of the committee to revise the breed Standard and the video committee.

ZOLLER, ROBERT J. While serving as a junior officer in the navy during World War II, Robert Zoller saw his first Alaskan Malamute. Zoller saw service in both the Atlantic and Pacific and ended up as a commander. At the end of the war he remained in the reserves. However, he never forgot the Alaskan Malamute he saw.

He was one of the founders of the Alaskan Malamute Club of America, serving as its president and for some years, edited and produced the news-letter that brought fanciers together.

He combined two strains of Arctic origin, and in the five years from 1953 to 1957 his Husky-Pak Malamutes won in every National Specialty competition in which they competed. His dogs were the foundation of many of the important Alaskan Malamute kennels active today.

About the Author

CONNIE VANACORE is an award-winning author and columnist with five published books and hundreds of columns about all aspects of the canine world and the sport of dogs to her credit. She wrote the section on dogs for the 1994 edition of *Encyclopedia Britannica* and has monthly columns in the dog press throughout the United States and Canada.

She has bred and owned Irish Setters since 1956, when she and her husband, Fred, purchased their first dog together. She has always owned a dog, her first being a Maltese purchased for her by her grandfather when she was two years old.

Connie is a past-president of the Irish Setter Club of America and of the Eastern Irish Setter Association. She is the founder and chairperson of the Irish Setter Club of America Health Committee and has enabled the national club to be in the forefront of fanciers supporting canine health research. She is an AKC delegate representing the Hollywood Dog Obedience Club, and is a member of the Delegates' Health Committee.

She has been a show chairperson for the Irish Setter Club of America National Specialty and for several local Specialties over the years, and she has held almost every office and been a member of the Board of Directors of her local and national club. She is a member of Somerset Hills Kennel Club (New Jersey).

She and her husband have two children and four grandchildren and divide their time between Mendham, New Jersey and Long Lake, New York, where they and their dogs spend the summers.

Connie enjoys travel and her collection of wildlife art and bronzes.

Index